# No Such Thing as Incurable

*A journey to self-healing made easy*

by

Annemarie St. Michael

## *Annemarie St. Michael*
### Registered Hypnotherapist and Health Educator
### Angels to the Rescue, LLC

---

## Important Cautions to the Reader

This book is not intended to diagnose any condition or disease, provide specific medical or other professional advice, or promote the sale of any product or service. None of the information or suggestions in this book should be used without first consulting a medical doctor and obtaining the doctor's consent to do so.

This book is sold on the condition and with the reader's understanding and agreement that the author and publisher shall not be liable or responsible for any damage, injury or loss alleged to be caused, directly or indirectly, by the information and suggestions contained in this book.

ISBN 978-0-9790549-0-7
First Edition

Printed in the United States of America

Published by Angels to the Rescue, LLC
       P.O. Box 2131
       Bonita Springs, FL 34135
       Toll Free: 866-9Angels
       www.angelstotherescue.com
       www.nosuchthingasincurable.com
       www.selfhealingmadeeasy.com

# Other Works by Annemarie St. Michael

*No Such Thing as Incurable Visualizations* - available in a two CD set containing eight healing visualizations.

*No Such Thing as Incurable Arthritis* - includes one CD with two healing visualizations

*Messages* - music CD

To order any of the above and this current book go to:

**www. SelfHealingMadeEasy.com** **or call 1-866-9Angels**

# Dedication

To my beloved friend, mentor and spiritual brother, Fletcher Johnston, whose patience, kindness and support taught me the true meaning of unconditional love.

# Acknowledgements

Without the time, love and assistance of the following, these ideas could never have been joyously set on these pages.

To my mom Mary Occhiuzzo, my greatest teacher, whose sacrifice, dedicated work ethic and generous nature molded me into the caring spirit I have become today.

To my family – Michael T. Sklaruk, Michael J. Sklaruk, Christopher Sklaruk, Christopher and Kassandra Smith, Rose Errico, Rita Borsilli, John and Effie Borsilli and Evalyn Errico, who allowed me to play teacher and whose loving support kept the dream alive.

To Jill Lawrence, my best friend and editor who worked tirelessly to keep me on track and whose unconditional love, sense of humor and incredible talent helped me convert abstract concepts into pictures and understandable words.

To Lyn Post, my business advisor who was always there with a laugh and who put down on paper the financial plan needed to bring this work to the world.

To Ryan Ward, graphic artist extraordinaire, whose vision and talent brought our beautiful logo, album cover, house of well being chart and this book cover to life.

To the crew at Audiolab – Ken Faulkenberry, Josh Young and Lou Panzer whose amazing technical and musical ability created the loving environment that birthed the audio visualizations.

To Amanda Reid my photographer, whose fast shutter and incredible eye turned an everyday grandma into a beautiful cover girl.

To all my friends, especially the members of our *Circle of Light* online healing circle - your willingness to be of service to those in need of prayers inspires me to stand firm in compassion and spread love.

And to the angels known as the Masters of the Family of Light, whose inspiration, love, guidance, constant protection and beautiful words have sparked my mind, soothed my heart, lifted my soul, healed my body and encouraged my spirit to come forth in service to assist humanity.

I am simply a messenger. Love to All.

# Contents

# I ntroduction

## Better to be Healed than Cured

Have you ever had a conversation so powerful and so life changing that you can remember it word for word? I have had at least two in my lifetime and one occurred on a brisk fall afternoon in 1992. The phone rang. It was my OB-GYN's nurse calling to set up another appointment. I had been to the doctor a few weeks earlier for unusual breakthrough bleeding and discomfort in my lower abdomen. My doctor had performed some uncomfortable procedures. The results were in and his nurse was calling to insist I return to the office.

"Annemarie, you MUST come back in," she said. "Why? What do I have?" I asked. She said, "Your test results show Type II dysplasia." Not having a clue as to what dysplasia was, my mind immediately ran to "it must be some type of IUD backlash". I gathered my courage to finally ask, "What's the big deal? What is dysplasia?" Suddenly there was silence on the other end. I became terribly frightened.

"Peggy, what is dysplasia?" I demanded. After a long pause, there was the emergence of a shaking voice. "It's serious." Her words were barely audible. "What do you mean serious? How serious?" I countered. "Annemarie, you have cancer." She said as gently as she could.

The lump in my throat was so big I couldn't swallow. Nausea swept over me and my hands were shaking. "Is there a cure?" I queried. "You have to speak to the doctor. When can you come in?" she countered.

Not only was I terrified but also left with no information. The Internet superhighway was just being built but I didn't own a computer, nor was I ready to head to the library to find out how serious this really was. All I knew was that at that time cancer was incurable and that I had just gotten the worst news of my life. I did have a dictionary though. Webster's New Collegiate version succinctly defined "incurable" as not curable.

That's it? Not curable? Why not? While my doctor eventually explained there was a possible procedure of freeze drying my cervix, there were no guarantees it would be successful or that the cancer wouldn't return. I wanted more assurances than that. I set out to find the "cure", but Webster defined "cure" as "restored to health, soundness or normality; to bring about recovery from." That wasn't good enough. I could cure the dysplasia with a medical or surgical procedure but may never have a healthy reproductive system again. I wanted more. I wanted what anyone in my position wanted - to be completely healed and to live a normal, healthy life.

"Pull yourself together, Annemarie," I said to myself. "You've done this before. You've already self-healed rheumatic heart disease as a child, manic-depression and arthritis, just a couple of years ago and chronic fatigue syndrome that had been plaguing you for almost eight years. This is just another one of God's tests. Calm down and call your best friend

Unfortunately, I couldn't calm down. The fear was overwhelming. I was caught in the middle of the semantic game played by the medical community, who had given strange names to the various stages of the disease and to this day does not call cancer "cancer" until the cell growth reaches higher proportions and/or they no longer have a treatment. As I write this, I am aware that some readers might say that type II dysplasia is not "cancer" because of the semantic game and therefore attempt to negate my entire experience. To those readers I would simply like to point out that for the lay person it's pretty simple – you either have cancer cells multiplying in your body or you do not. The terror that I experienced for over four months was real indeed. I was going against doctor's orders on personal convictions and flying without a net. The abnormal cells could have easily spread to the higher stages. I could have lost my female organs and/or died. Had any of that taken place, I would not be here today to assist others who might also be suffering the extreme emotional fear associated with such a diagnosis.

I did not make the appointment for the freezing procedure since I decided to risk all or nothing on my former natural treatments. I immediately picked up the phone and made the call to one of my dear friends who was also a gifted spiritual teacher and healing instrument. Through her I might be able to get the information I needed to turn the emerging cancer around.

First she gave me the name an herbalist in California who was a naturopath and had developed a line of herbal products. I immediately called him and ordered the formulas he suggested I take to calm the cancer growth while rebuilding and strengthening the immune system and the female organs.

Then I sat down with one of my spiritual teachers, who gave me the dietary protocol that I am sharing with you on the subsequent pages that would help me complete a full body detox. In addition, they suggested I schedule a colonic once a week for the next five weeks to clear out any accumulated debris in my system and allow the body to absorb more nourishment, which it needed in order to reverse the condition. They also suggested I keep a daily log of everything, including my food choices and all the herbals and supplements I was ingesting. Recording every event that was taking place into a journal was another suggestion that they gave me. With such a useful tool, I could easily watch my progress and be encouraged to stay on track until the cancer was gone.

They then gave the most important piece of advice by suggesting that I do daily visualizations differently. "To completely heal your body, you must heal the emotional root," they advised. "How do I do that and how will I know when it's over," I asked. "You will be intuitively and angelically guided if you ask for help. Then you will go back to the doctor for another examination and be tested again. When your doctor tells you he has received the documented proof that your tests are negative, your mind will be finally put to rest and it will be over," was the response.

While I don't advocate going against doctor's advice, I was in a different position than most people. I had already healed four so-called incurable illnesses and had a good track record with herbals and natural remedies. I was confident and leaned toward the holistic approach to healing. I was ready, willing and able to take it on. However, what I learned through the experience brought me to a new level of understanding that I would never have achieved had it not occurred. I realized during the process that being diagnosed with type II dysplasia was the greatest gift that my Creator could have given me.

Armed only with the love and direction of my teachers, I took all the principles I had learned from Christianity to Hebrew Kaballah to modern day spiritualism and put them all into full practice. For almost four months I cleansed and renewed my body, mind, emotions and spirit. I learned through my visualizations that we are all connected and that we are part of our Creator and He/She is a part of us. Since what most of us call "God" cannot be sick, cannot be broke and cannot be dead, we who were made in the "image and likeness" are the same. We only think we are sick, broke or dead and therefore unknowingly create the experience for ourselves through our thoughts, beliefs and subsequent actions.

I also learned that in an effort to experience that specific all-important universal truth, sometimes we are challenged with illness so we have an opportunity to clean up our act. In so doing not only do we advance our soul's journey to become more connected to our Creator, we are sometimes also offered an opportunity to leave the planet through our illness as well. Oftentimes we are finished here on earth and have other business to perform on the other side. Illness is not a punishment and death is simply the "spiritual healing" or opportunity to sometimes shed a sick body for a beautiful new body of light so that we can continue to be of service to one another from the different realms many of us call heaven.

A great teacher by the name of Abraham explains that we go from pure positive physical energy to pure positive non-physical energy. We are always alive and healthy somewhere. Either here or on the other side, which I like to think of as being "out of town". Our own soul decides and makes the choice without the consent of our conscious mind. There is no person or no circumstance to blame. Everything always occurs in *Divine Right Order*. There is always a reason and our soul choices are part of the equation.

While soul choices may be responsible for bringing on certain experiences, it is our conscious choices that alter our attitude as a result of those circumstances. Ultimately, attitude directs the quality of our lives.

We can clearly see those principles at work in the story of the somewhat bigoted Samaritan woman who met Jesus at Jacob's well supposedly by accident. At first the woman was challenged to give water to a Jew who in her belief was someone to avoid. However, after he gives her a reading of her past and present living situation and uses the water analogy to suggest she look elsewhere to re-establish her spiritual connection, she becomes hopeful and makes a choice to shift her prejudicial thinking and changes her attitude. With a renewed spirit she leaves her water jar and goes back to her town to invite her neighbors to check out the man whose insights had just rocked her world. Eventually she and many of her fellow Samaritans close the prejudicial gap by embracing the messages that cured their attitude.

Those of us who are experiencing life with physical or emotional handicaps might consider following her example and adopt an "attitudinal healing." While there may not be a "physical cure" for a maimed or handicapped physical body, there is surely an "attitudinal healing" that can shift the mind and spirit and heal the emotional body of its wounds to help you live with whatever physical restrictions you have. Learning to be happy and as healthy as one can be, even in the face of handicaps, is the "healing" for a soul who has chosen the bodily status quo for a more difficult earthly experience that can offer more wisdom and compassion.

For some who are experiencing mental challenges, there may be hope in herbal and dietary remedies and in outside stimuli that can trigger the brain back into normal function e.g. exercise, music, art, handicrafts can all be related to "physical healings." Some may also experience an "attitudinal healing" while under the influence of pharmaceuticals or in therapy and sometimes by using creative visualization techniques and/or prayer. Other mental sufferers might appear to be incurable because they are experiencing a soul choice or pre-written script they crafted prior to incarnating to be of service to humanity by being institutionalized thus allowing those around them to become caregivers before they themselves achieve their "spiritual healing."

This brings me to another truth that was revealed to me through my health challenges. From the defining moment of the nurse's phone call, I was no longer a working mom worrying about school, laundry and the demands of my career, but a seriously ill mom who was thrust into a battle for her life. Just like many of us who are pushed beyond our limit and have nowhere to turn, I made a deal with God that day. I promised that if He or She could help me find the steps to heal completely, I would focus all of my energy on the task and do whatever it took to stay on the planet and take care of my family.

With the full knowledge of my entire being that there is no death, only transition, came the revelation that there are at least three levels of healings for every situation – physical, attitudinal and spiritual. Armed with such a powerful insight, I then vowed to metaphorically climb to the highest building and shout from the rooftop "If I can heal myself so can you. There is no such thing as incurable!"

# Chapter 1

# Are you ready to be healed?

## Medical View

In order to plan any trip, we need to know our destination. In this case, I would like to suggest that being healed would be our goal or our destination. But for us to reach that destination, we need to define exactly what the word "healed" means. According to my 1973 Webster's New Collegiate Dictionary, the definition of "healed" is: "The condition of being sound in body, mind and spirit; to make whole." That was a pretty enlightened statement for Webster as far back as 1973. The question is, now that we understand where we are going, how do we get there? Well, that can be simple, too. First, we need to take a look at where we are and, more importantly, how we got here.

When scientists look at our physical ailments, they only look in one place—the physical body. They contend that although emotional factors may accentuate the problem, for the most part, sickness starts somewhere in the physical body as brought about by one or more of five common causes: Hereditary, Invasive Organisms, Exposure, Trauma, or Poor Diet.

**Heredity** is the scientists' reference to our genes or DNA, and that usually includes things like birth defects and inherited tendencies.

**Invasive Organisms** are the most common causes of illness and these are the ones scientists look for first: Virus, Bacteria, Fungus, and Parasites. Scientists spend billions of dollars each year trying to isolate these organisms in order to heal us. Sometimes they are successful, but many articles have been published lately that tell us that these organisms continually mutate, and the drugs sometimes wind up having no effect on the new strains.

**Exposure** is another common cause of illness. We are exposed to various types of climate changes, to chemicals in our water and food, pollutants in our air, and toxic electromagnetic fields that can wreak havoc on our brain and body waves. All of these types of exposures can be traced to several diseases, especially allergies and bronchial congestion.

**Trauma** can be divided into two categories: Physical Trauma and Emotional Trauma.

*Physical Trauma* is easy to identify because it usually involves an accident of some kind. Suppose you fall down and break your leg necessitating the need for crutches to move around. Without realizing what you are doing, placing more weight onto your wrists and arms to support your body may knock them out of alignment. Years later, this act may result in a wearing down of the joints leading to Arthritis. It can also lead to torn muscles, which can in turn lead to scar tissue.

*Emotional Trauma* can be the most severe. Have you ever seen a horrible accident or a murder? Some people have actually gone into a catatonic state for years after witnessing something terrible. When soldiers come home from a war, oftentimes they experience what used to be called "shell shock," but that too has a fancy new name: Now they call it "post-war traumatic syndrome" or "post-traumatic stress disorder." Many veterans have nightmares, become very nervous, and develop all kinds of illnesses.

**Poor Diet** is also a contributing factor to illness. We don't pay enough attention to our diet because here in America, food is abundant and we have virtually wiped out the diseases like scurvy and beriberi. However, there is so much confusion about the role diet plays in the creation of our sickness as well as in the healing process. Lately, Poor Diet also has been the catchall for everything from Diabetes and Heart disease to Athlete's Foot. There has been so much written on proper diet that we're all swimming with more information than we can handle. The worst part is that the information changes every week, according to which book or magazine you pick up. I think that Susan Powter is right when she says that we need to "stop the insanity." We've all gone over the edge.

And lastly there is the elusive sixth cause of disease. Now this one shouldn't have a bullet because it doesn't really exist. It's the **"I don't know where it came from"** category. Haven't you noticed that most diseases fall into that one? The frustration of not knowing the source of your illness or how to stop it from progressing is the most difficult part for most people to overcome. You can end up going for a ride on the Fear roller coaster with little hope in sight. Invasive procedures, while sometimes necessary, leave us wounded and without recourse. And the silent side effect of liver dysfunction, which comes with many drugs, does not make for long-term solutions.

I invite you to take a look at another possibility. As the following illustrations suggest, I discovered that we don't just have a physical body as seen in diagram number one; we also have a mental body, an emotional body and a spiritual body.

# Our Four Bodies

**1) Physical Body**

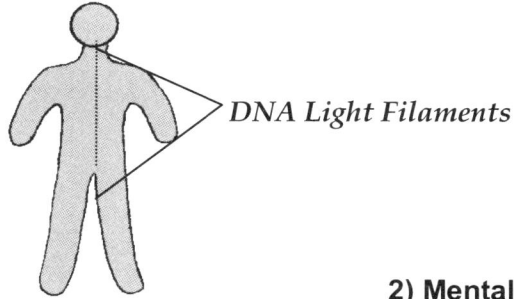

*DNA Light Filaments*

**2) Mental Body**
*Home of the Ego*

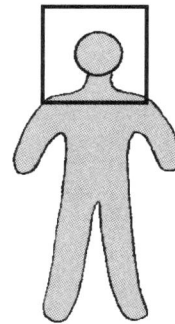

**3) Emotional Body**

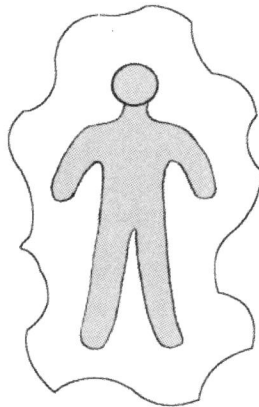

**4) Spiritual Body**

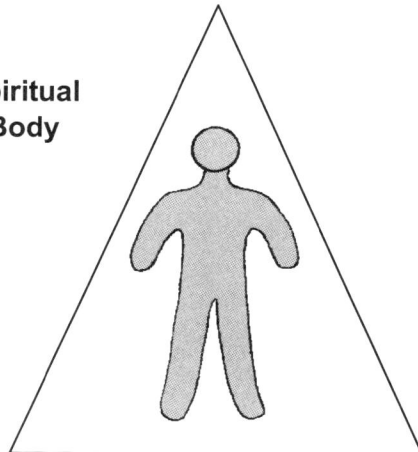

The mental body is the home of the ego personality, which I have represented as a square in diagram number two because ego mind is the seat of fear and always attempts to back us into a corner. The emotional body, as indicated in diagram number three, never stays in one place so I used wavy lines to represent the highs and lows that are typical of human emotions. And lastly, in diagram number four, I chose the pyramid for the spiritual body, which to me represents the three aspects of all life, including the three aspects of humankind: body, mind and spirit.

If we go back to our original definition of being healed as "sound in body, mind and spirit," it seems clear to me that our scientists are overlooking the obvious: They are not addressing all four bodies. Maybe the reason that our scientists cannot find the answers to curing chronic diseases by taking apart the physical body is because the illness didn't start there in the first place.

If you look at diagram number one, the small dots represent our DNA light filaments that run up and down our spinal column. The scientists tell us that every cell in our body is encoded with our own unique DNA signature— sort of like a fingerprint. It's the blueprint that decided our hair color, our skin color, our bone structure, blood type, and all the deciding factors that make each of us different. Scientists also tell us that the body is made up of cells, and within the cells are atoms. These atoms are made up of protons, neutrons and electrons, all of which are stored energy charges. If we split the atoms, we have a powerful energy source.

Follow this for a moment: If you were to place your hand under a very powerful microscope, not only would you see the cells and their atoms, but you would also see the empty space between them. According to Dr. Deepak Chopra, in his book "Ageless Body, Timeless Mind," this void makes up over 70% of our body. We are mostly empty space! No wonder so many of us float through life without a clue!

Basically, we are a loosely formed clump made up of specks of energy in constant motion, floating in space with its own intelligence.  In simple layman's terms, we are made up of only two things: Energy and Consciousness.  The Consciousness creates, and the Energy moves that creation into being.  I wonder how many of us heard that before?  In Sunday school maybe?

If our scientists don't know what truly causes disease, and our spiritual leaders don't know, and the tribal shamans don't know, then who does?  Well, I can only think of one Being.  A Being that is All knowing, All loving, Everywhere, All powerful, All creation, All diverse, and comes in All varieties.    You know whom I mean.    The omniscient, omnipresent, omnipotent, omnificent and omnifarious God, sometimes called God / Goddess / All That Is / Universal Energy / Infinite One / Beloved Parent / Creator.  It doesn't matter what name you choose.  For our purposes, we'll be using either God/Goddess or Creator.  I know that thinking of God in the feminine is difficult for some of us, however about a year ago even the Southern Baptist Convention decided to remove all the masculine biblical references of God and somehow present God as gender neutral.  I myself have come to believe that the being we call God is not either masculine or feminine but more of an endomorph - a he/she if you will, encompassing the best attributes of both.    In deep visualization I was given that the most politically correct title could be God/Goddess/All That Is.

My Sunday school teacher taught me that we were made in the image and likeness of our Creator.  Wouldn't that mean that He/She is also made up of the same Energy and Consciousness?  If our Creator is everywhere, aren't we part of everywhere?  What about being omnifarious?  That means being all varieties, like a bird, a tree, a rock, a waterfall.  If animals are a variety of Creator, what about humans?

If we are to believe that Creator is everywhere, in all varieties, then what is wrong with the following illustration?

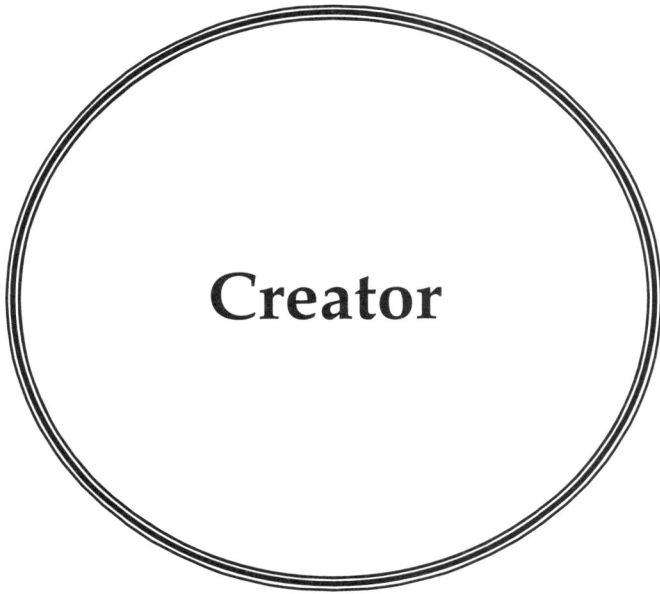

**Creator**

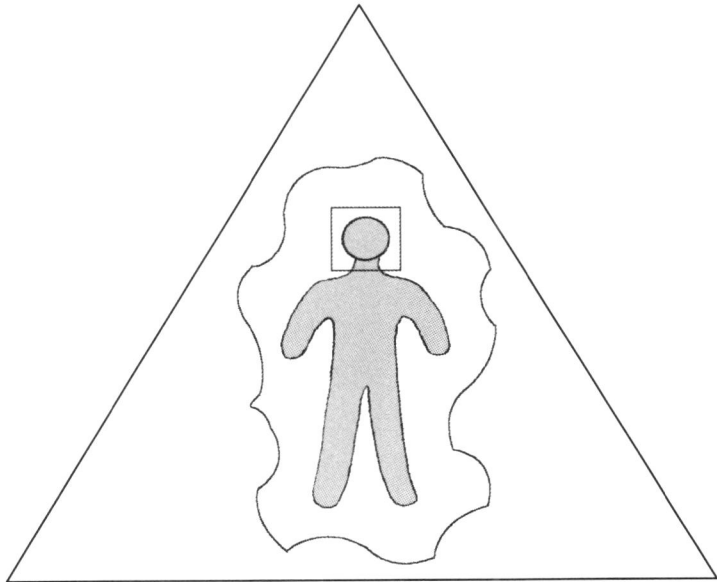

I have come to believe it is actually more like this:

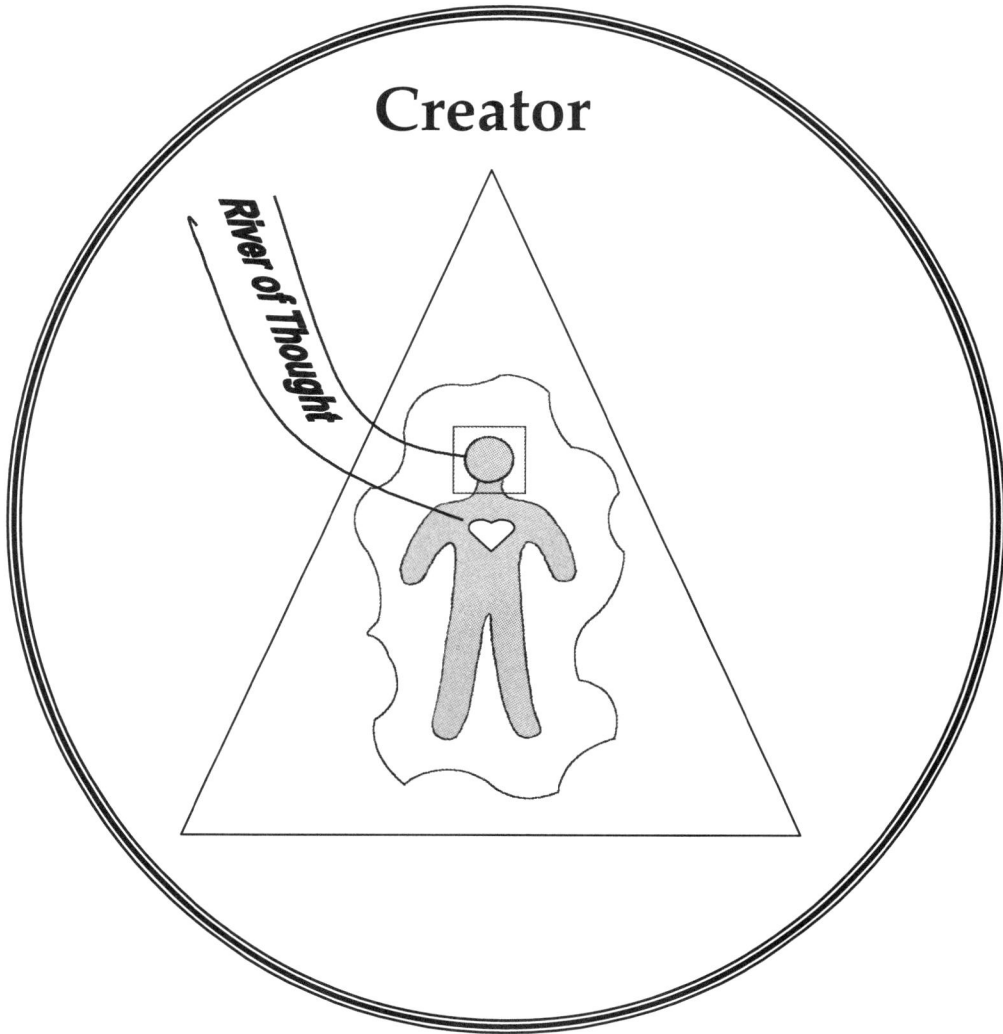

# Creator

**River of Thought**

I don't expect you to take my word for it. This work was designed for you to discover your own truth. Right now, you are holding in your hands an opportunity to discover whether this connection exists or not. I call it the "River of Thought. " It's a channel or passageway for an exchange of information. I believe that it is part of the biblical promise: "Before you call, I will answer," and is directly connected like a "y" cable from our Creator to our heart and to the top of our head.

I once heard a great spiritual teacher by the name of Ramtha say that behind our heart is a cavity wherein lies our soul, our direct link to our Creator. First I thought it was strange, but now I understand. Like Neale Donald Walsch in his books *Conversations with God*, I too plugged in and simply asked. Since our soul knows only one thing, and that is unconditional love, I decided to call it our Love Essence. In that way, we are reminded of who we truly are.

Our Love Essence is also the home of what some call the "Voice of the Holy Spirit." I like to call it my Higher Wisdom, because it is wiser than my normal reasoning and only speaks truth. It's that tiny voice within, which is more like a feeling that we then translate into words in our brain. It comes from Creator, then travels from heart to head, and completes the Y-connection back to Creator. Our Love Essence is also the place where our Creator and we co-exist as a team, working together to continually create. When we are not in the state of Love, our team captain reminds us it is time to get back on track by knocking on one or more of our seven major energy centers and creating an imbalance. It's like Creator saying, "Hello, it's time to forgive your brother-in-law for the $500 he borrowed from you ten years ago and never paid back," or something like that.

In my experience, all the symptoms and pain that we experience in our state of dis-ease is actually our Higher Wisdom speaking to us. The sickness itself **IS** the communication. Again, without sounding too crazy, it's a gift from God to let us know that we are not paying attention to our soul's work.

It is up to us to interpret what the illness is saying to us. When we finally figure it out and take care of it, the sickness has done its job and we don't need it anymore.

As an example, if you're feeling hot and you see something red or swollen, you probably have been holding onto some type of anger for too long. If you are cold or blue, you may be experiencing sadness or a hidden feeling of guilt. If your illness causes palpitations, you can bet your last quarter that it is a stress signal resulting from either a known or an unknown fear.

Here's the good news. When you learn to quiet the intellectual mind and to listen very carefully to your Higher Wisdom, you too can get to those root messages. It takes a little practice, but all of my students have been able to get through eventually. I have a perfect record and I'm counting on you to help me keep it. Learning to tap in is the first, the biggest, and the hardest step in your healing process, but you don't have to do it alone. I've practically done it for you and I'll be with you every step of the way.

**Types of Prayers**

❖ Supplication - " Creator/God/Goddess please help me…"

❖ Gratitude - "Thank you Creator/God/Goddess for…"

❖ Affirmations - "I am…"

❖ Action/Creation - "I intend to…(or) I choose to create…"

❖ Surrender - "I release…for the highest and best good of all. "

Since we were little, almost all of us have been told that we could bridge the gap to our Creator through prayer. Praying was the number one method of choice for communication but most of those prayers were prayers of supplication(s), as you can see. You know the kind—when we ask for something like, "Please, God, send me a new pair of roller skates." Then there were the bargaining prayers: "God, if you could only get me a date with Donald Duck, I promise to go to church every Sunday for the rest of my life. Amen. "

Then, of course, we learned our prayers of gratitude, especially around Thanksgiving time. Now, it's easy to say "thank you" when you're staring at a beautifully stuffed turkey on your table. But what about saying "thank you" for your turkey dinner on the night before Thanksgiving, when you're broke, out of a job, the fridge is empty, and you have no clue how you're going to put food on that table. That's what enlightenment calls us to do. To say "thank you" for something that hasn't arrived yet. That is putting the "faith of the mustard seed" into practice. But it is more than an act of faith. If you truly believe that somehow a holiday dinner will miraculously appear, it becomes an act of trust and there's a world of difference between the two.

Faith to me is kind of a wishy-washy word. Most of us have faith in a power that is greater than our own, or faith in another's capabilities but believing that that power will come through for us in the nick of time, that's a horse of a different color. Saying you believe in God is an act of *faith*, but closing your eyes, crossing your hands on your chest, and falling backward, knowing that God will catch you—now that is a complete act of *trust*.

The reason I chose prayers of gratitude for your visualizations was because my Higher Wisdom said that it was the greatest gift that we could give to ourselves. That in the acceptance of Love in gratitude we actually halt the disease process and start healing. Stay in *trust* and watch miracles happen in your life.

There are two other types of prayers that I've used in this program with which you may or may not be familiar. One is a prayer of power, usually called an affirmation. Those prayers always start with the words "I Am. " They affirm your belief that you are in partnership with God, and that you have some say in the matter. They are the most powerful prayers we can say, provided our *trust* is intact.

The other type of prayer may be new to you. It's a little softer than an affirmation, and great for flexing your new spiritual muscles. It's called a prayer of action. It starts with the words "I intend to," or "I command," or "I call forth." It sort of sets the stage for something great to happen.

## Creator Talks Back

Since we all know how to talk to Creator, it begs the question: "How does Creator talk to us?" Well, there are many ways that our Creator uses to speak to us. Again, going back to "God is everywhere and in all varieties," that could mean that Creator speaks to us through other people. Have you ever had the experience of being at your wits' end while trying to make a decision or find something, when out of nowhere; a friend or a total stranger offered some simple advice that solved your problem?

What about Creator speaking to us through a book? That could be any or every book. It was my reading and listening to "Conversations with God" by Neale Donald Walsch that gave me the final piece to this work. When you're ready for some major revelations, I suggest that you read it, too or better still, get the tapes. They are awesome and you can listen to them over and over again.

Another way that Creator can talk to us is through our dreams. Many of us have gotten warnings about certain events in our dream state. It's a very common occurrence. Moses himself talked to the Burning Bush, but the voice that came back was his own, speaking in his own mind. If you don't believe me, just ask Charlton Heston.

All kidding aside, the most difficult communication between Creator and us is through our sickness. Oh, I know that's a tough one, but the idea of God talking to us through our sickness is not such a crazy notion if we understand how we're connected and how the energy in our body flows.

Turn to page 20 and check out the Chakra Locations and Symbols illustration. As you can see, our chakra lady has seven major energy centers. The bible refers to them as the lamp stands, but in ancient Sanskrit they were called the "chakras," which means "wheels of energy. " The first is located at the base of the spine, and it is responsible for all our creativity including ideas, works of art and of course, procreation. When it is balanced, we are active, alive, and in a creative mode.

The second chakra is located mid-abdomen and is called the pelvic chakra. It helps keep us centered and calm. The third is called the solar plexus chakra and is located in the middle of our stomach. It is usually the place we call our "gut feeling." It warns us of danger and is sometimes called our second brain.

The fourth chakra is located just above our heart. As you would expect, it is our center of love; however, it is commonly knocked out of balance by anxiety, which in turn causes an imbalance in our natural hormone flow. It's what the doctors call "the stress response."

The fifth chakra is located at the base of our throat and is responsible for both our verbal and telepathic communication and our ability to swallow nourishment. The sixth chakra is located in the middle of our forehead, and is called the "brow chakra" or the "third eye chakra. " It helps us to see beyond the physical planes into the higher realms.

And finally, the seventh chakra is located at the top of our head and is called the "crown chakra." It is responsible for higher brain functions and is the doorway to the spiritual realms. It is through the crown chakra that we enter and exit our bodies every night and morning. Think of it as a dimmer switch. When you turn down the juice, you dim the lights. That's what we do everyday when we go to sleep. We let out most of our energy so that the body can rest. When the body has had enough rest, we crawl back in again. Have you ever woken up suddenly and felt like you had crash-landed? That's because your consciousness re-entered the body too fast. When all our energy centers are purring along nicely, we are healthy, balanced and at ease. When they are out of balance, all the organs and systems under their control become unhealthy and eventually diseased. The question is: "What knocks them out?"

## Understanding Dis-Ease

For that answer, we need to look into the consciousness of the body part that is at the point of pain or dis-ease. A few years ago, every morning I woke up with a backache. Thinking it was time to chuck out my old mattress, I spent $400 on a new one before I finally asked my back what was wrong. I had to chuckle when it told me that all it wanted me to do was to take a hot shower before I went to my yoga class to warm up my muscles. When I complied, the pain stopped immediately.

The next places we need to examine are the mental and emotional bodies. In my experience, nearly every time I communicated with my Higher Wisdom, my head and my heart were at war. There was always an old hurt that needed to be healed. It could have been a recent incident or one that had occurred maybe 10 or 20 years ago. For whatever reason, the hurt had not been resolved. All the anger, frustration, disappointment, fears, and guilt somehow got tied into a knot. When I was able to untie the knot, the sickness, whatever it was, started to turn around and I could easily get a handle on it. When I followed up with good nutrition and herbal support, eventually the illness left me forever.

To become whole, as Webster has suggested, we need to re-balance our chakras. There is only one thing that can re-balance and heal our body, and that is Love. I've come to believe that "Love is the Answer" is more than just a song. It is a universal truth. Without it, we literally self-destruct. When we can find it in our heart to forgive those who have hurt us and include ourselves in that act of forgiving, we are well on our way to healing even the most serious illness.

As I've said before, praying is speaking to our Creator, but very few of us in the western hemisphere have been taught to listen. To listen, you must quiet the intellectual body because as I said before, it is the home of the ego. Someone once very appropriately said that ego stands for "Edge God Out. " But it is even more than that. Ego is our voice of judgment. It is the conversation held within our head that says something like, "Could you believe how she is behaving? I wouldn't be caught dead doing that. " It is also the voice of fear that separates us from each other, and the call of despair in the middle of the night. Like, "If I don't get a job soon, how will I pay the mortgage? There's no one to help me. " Ego is the irrational belief that we can do everything without godly assistance. "I can figure it out. I'll have to do a little maneuvering here and there, but I know exactly how it will go down. " It's also the voice of the bully that fosters bigotry and hatred. "Who do they think they are, moving in here? I'll fix them!"

But the ego isn't all bad. It's also the voice that says, "Hey, don't play in traffic—you're liable to get hurt!" Ego is just part of our earthly experience and we have to deal with it. An easy way to stop the chatter is simply to say to the ego, "Mind be still and know that I am love," then wait for the silence.

# Chapter 2

## How to Heal Completely

### 8 Steps to Healing

B   Befriend Your Illness

E   Eliminate Pain

H   Hear the Message

E   Evaluate Your Illness

A   Absolve (cleanse) all
    four Bodies

L   Line up physical
    assistance

E   Execute Your Program

D   Declare Thanks to
    Creator

### Step 1:  Letter "B" - Befriend your Illness

It's as simple as the words "Be Healed." Now let's pretend for a minute that you just cut your finger in the kitchen. The first thing that you do is the "B," which stands for Befriend your illness. Now what do I mean by that? I mean stop fighting. Do you make war on your cut finger by hating it? Of course not, you simply know that it's a cut and immediately spring into action. You don't go around screaming, "Oh my God, I'll never play the violin again!" Do you? Then why do we go crazy when we are given a difficult diagnosis?

For as long as I can remember, we have always used war metaphors when we talk about eliminating illness. We say things like, "We're gonna fight this thing," or "We've added a new drug to our arsenal of weapons to fight…"

17

Think for a minute. Isn't the illness part of your body? Hasn't it taken up residence there? If you go to war against your own body please tell me who loses? That's right, you do! So, how do you stop a war? Simple—lay down your weapons. The best way to halt an illness in its tracks is to pull the plug on its power over you. Make friends with it. Love it. It's not some evil plague that a merciless deity vested on you. It's an opportunity. In some ways, it's an opportunity to test your metal, to learn how to heal and to discover who you really are. So make friends with it. Thank it for coming into your life as a teacher. Tell it that you are sorry for not acknowledging your part in bringing it about. Vow to do better by listening to your body more carefully. When you honor your illness with that kind of Love, it has done the job of reaching you, and will only hang around if you don't keep your word and make the necessary changes for the healing to take place.

## Step 2:  Letter "E" -  Eliminate Pain

The next thing that you probably did when you cut your finger was to yell "OW. " That brings us to our next letter, "E": Eliminate Pain. With a cut, you can put ice on it or run it under cold water, but when the pain is internal it becomes kind of tricky. You can either take what you usually take to bring down the pain level, or try to bring it down with your mind. Pain is merely a signal from the brain to tell us that something is wrong.

I remember being stuck once in the middle of nowhere forest in north Florida at least forty miles from civilization. I suddenly got struck with the worst headache I ever had. All I could do was pull over, massage my temples and focus on some prayers. I didn't even know how to visualize at the time. When I focused on the prayers, the pain got short-circuited, and in less than ten minutes, it was gone and I was able to get back behind the wheel. Now that's power—the ability to move mind over pain. Anyone can do it, if they practice.

The  other  most important  reason  to  eliminate  the pain  is not just for

# Chakra Locations and Symbols

**7 - Crown chakra**
    Color - Violet
    Pineal Gland
    Energy Intake and Connection to Source

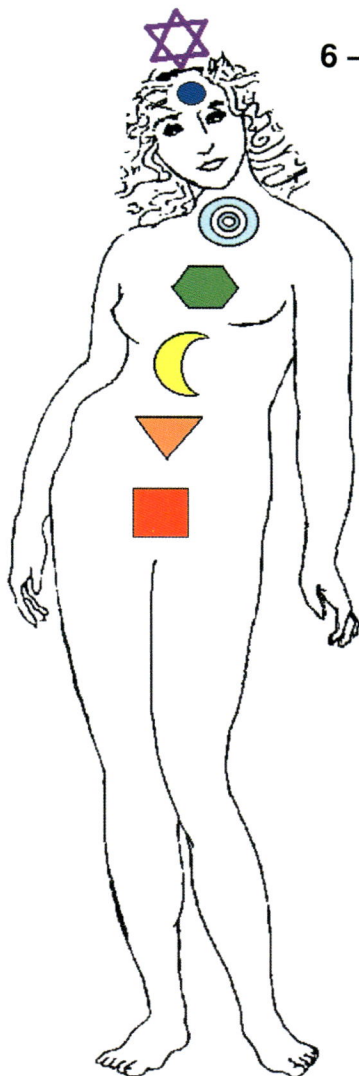

**6 – Third Eye (Brow) chakra**
    Color – Indigo
    Pituitary Gland
    The ability to bring past and future into the present

**5 –Throat chakra**
    Turquoise
    Center of Communication and Telepathy

**4 - Heart chakra**
    Color - Grass Green
    Thymus Gland
    Center of our Soul

**3 – Solar plexus chakra**
    Color – Yellow
    Adrenal Glands
    Center of Intuitive Feeling

**2 – Pelvic chakra**
    Color – Orange
    Center of the Emotional Body

**1 – Root chakra**
    Color – Red

19

# Chakra Symbol Chart

| Location/Function | Symbol | Color/ Balancing Color | Musical Note |
|---|---|---|---|
| 1) Root Chakra *Center of Creativity* | Square | Red/Kelly Green | C – Doe |
| 2) Pelvic Chakra *Center of Emotional Body and Serenity* | Inverted Triangle | Orange/ Yellow Orange | E – Me |
| 3) Solar Plexus Chakra *Center of Intuitive Feeling* | Quarter Moon | Yellow/Off White | D – Ray |
| 4) Heart Chakra *Center of Soul/Love* | Hexagon | Grass Green/Violet | F – Fa |
| 5) Throat Chakra *Center of Communication and Telepathy* | Concentric Circles | Turquoise/Sky Blue | G – So |
| 6) Brow Chakra (Third Eye) *Center of Inner Vision* | Dot | Indigo/Pink | A – La |
| 7) Crown Chakra *Center of Spirituality and Doorway to Source* | Star of David | Violet/Gold | B - Tea |

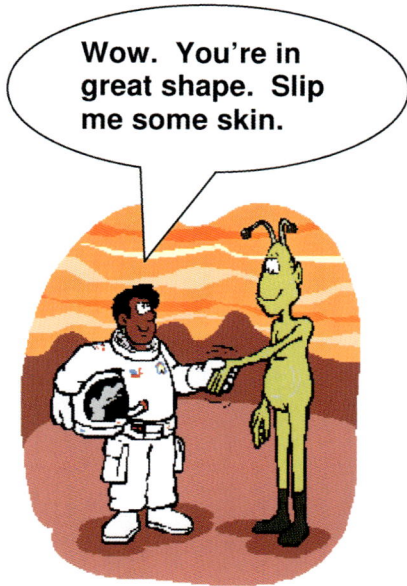

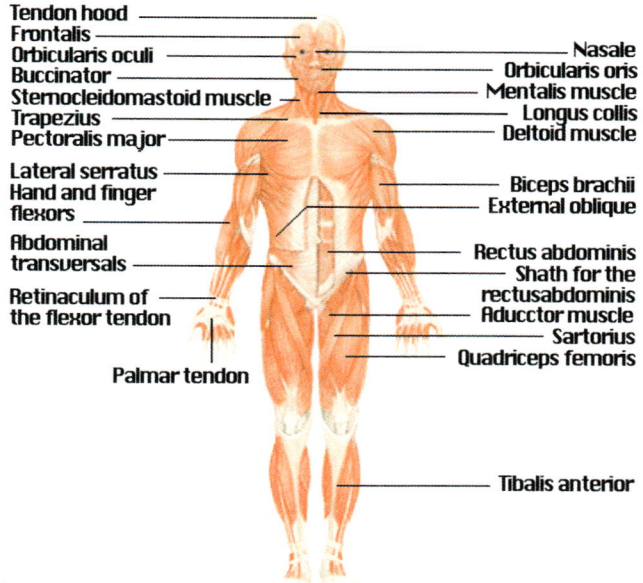

Tendon hood
Frontalis
Orbicularis oculi
Buccinator
Sternocleidomastoid muscle
Trapezius
Pectoralis major

Nasale
Orbicularis oris
Mentalis muscle
Longus collis
Deltoid muscle

Lateral serratus
Hand and finger flexors

Biceps brachii
External oblique

Abdominal transversals

Rectus abdominis
Shath for the rectusabdominis
Aducctor muscle
Sartorius
Quadriceps femoris

Retinaculum of the flexor tendon

Palmar tendon

Tibalis anterior

# Muscles-Back

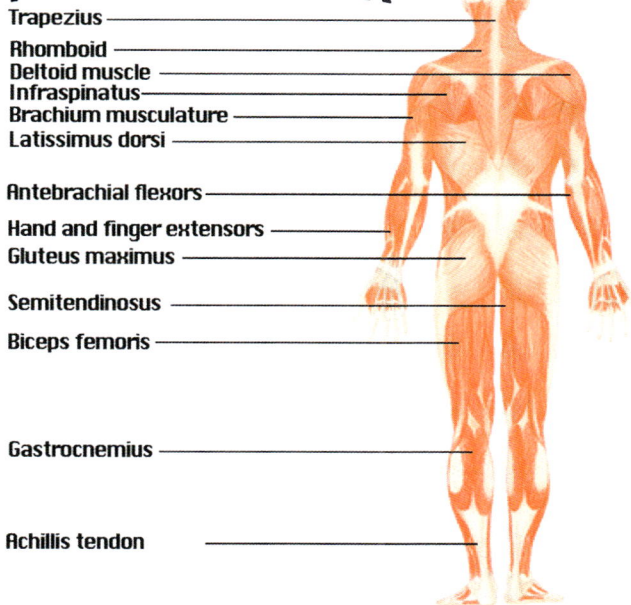

Trapezius

Rhomboid
Deltoid muscle
Infraspinatus
Brachium musculature
Latissimus dorsi

Antebrachial flexors

Hand and finger extensors
Gluteus maximus

Semitendinosus

Biceps femoris

Gastrocnemius

Achillis tendon

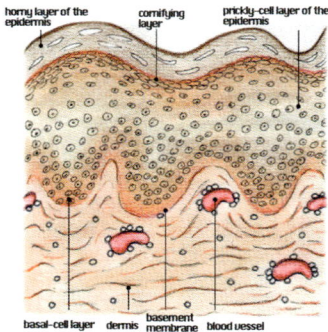

horny layer of the epidermis
cornifying layer
prickly-cell layer of the epidermis

basal-cell layer  dermis  basement membrane  blood vessel

# The Skin

Body Illustrations from Human 3D, Mega Systems, Duluth, GA    www.mega-systems.net

## Skeletal System

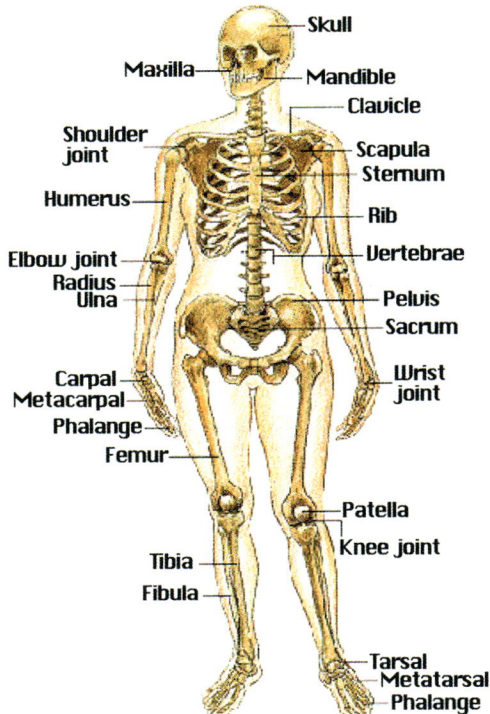

- Skull
- Maxilla
- Mandible
- Clavicle
- Shoulder joint
- Scapula
- Sternum
- Humerus
- Rib
- Elbow joint
- Vertebrae
- Radius
- Ulna
- Pelvis
- Sacrum
- Carpal
- Metacarpal
- Wrist joint
- Phalange
- Femur
- Patella
- Knee joint
- Tibia
- Fibula
- Tarsal
- Metatarsal
- Phalange

## Respiratory System

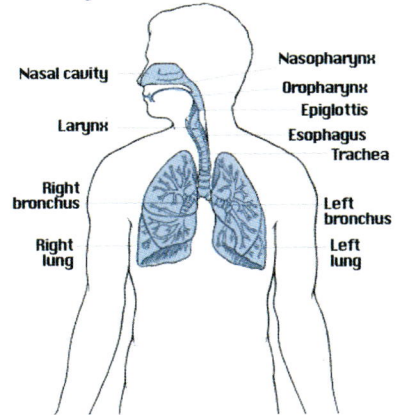

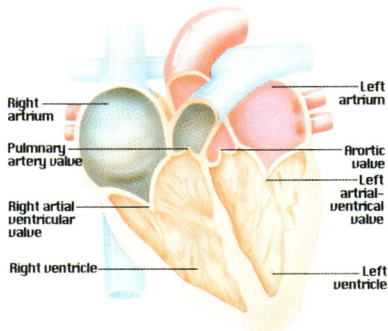

- Nasal cavity
- Nasopharynx
- Oropharynx
- Epiglottis
- Larynx
- Esophagus
- Trachea
- Right bronchus
- Left bronchus
- Right lung
- Left lung

## Heart Chambers

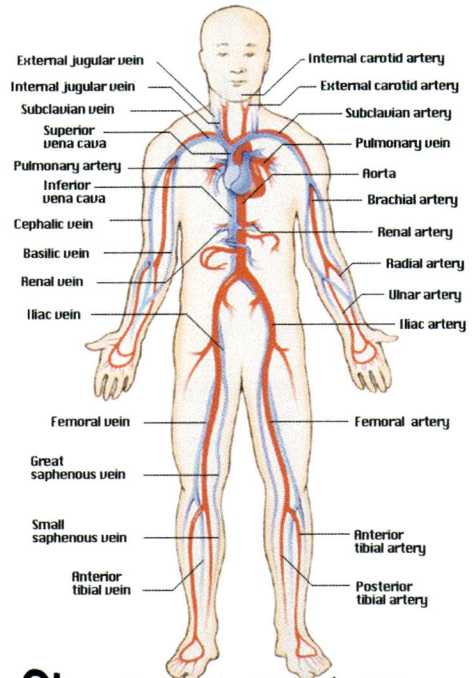

- Right atrium
- Left atrium
- Pulmnary artery valve
- Aortic valve
- Left atrial-ventrical valve
- Right artial ventricular valve
- Right ventricle
- Left ventricle

## Circulatory System

- External jugular vein
- Internal carotid artery
- Internal jugular vein
- External carotid artery
- Subclavian vein
- Subclavian artery
- Superior vena cava
- Pulmonary vein
- Pulmonary artery
- Aorta
- Inferior vena cava
- Brachial artery
- Cephalic vein
- Renal artery
- Basilic vein
- Radial artery
- Renal vein
- Ulnar artery
- Iliac vein
- Iliac artery
- Femoral vein
- Femoral artery
- Great saphenous vein
- Small saphenous vein
- Anterior tibial artery
- Anterior tibial vein
- Posterior tibial artery

Body Illustrations from Human 3D, Mega Systems, Duluth, GA    www.mega-systems.net

*How to Heal Completely*

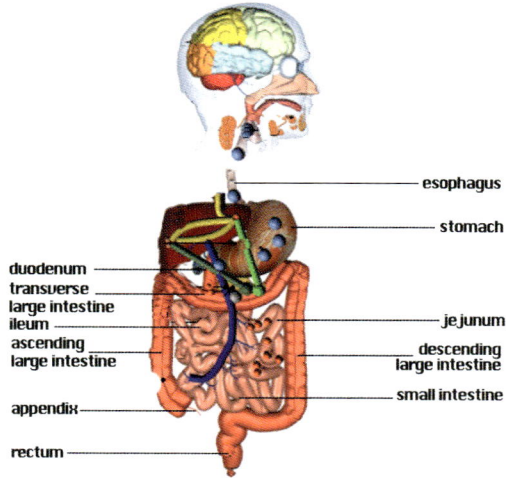

**Female Reproductive System**

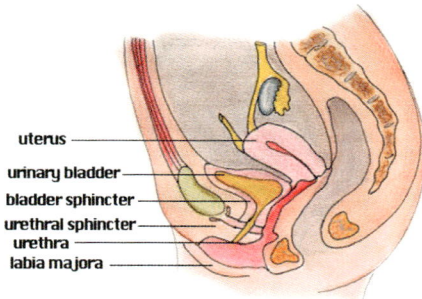

esophagus, stomach, duodenum, transverse large intestine, ileum, ascending large intestine, appendix, rectum, jejunum, descending large intestine, small intestine

**Let's Cha Cha Cha**

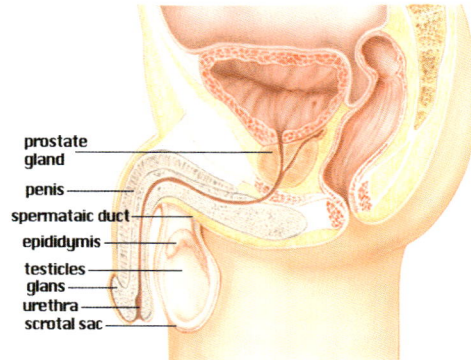

**Female Reproductive Organs**

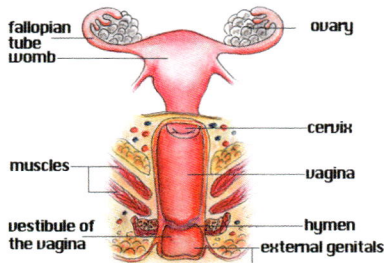

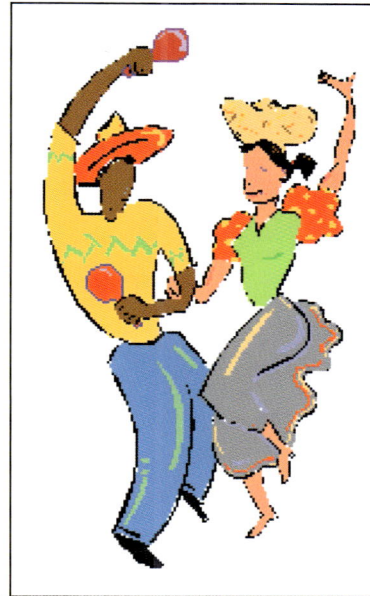

uterus, urinary bladder, bladder sphincter, urethral sphincter, urethra, labia majora

fallopian tube, womb, muscles, vestibule of the vagina, ovary, cervix, vagina, hymen, external genitals

**Male Reproductive System**

prostate gland, penis, spermataic duct, epididymis, testicles, glans, urethra, scrotal sac

Body Illustrations from Human 3D, Mega Systems, Duluth, GA    www.mega-systems.net

23

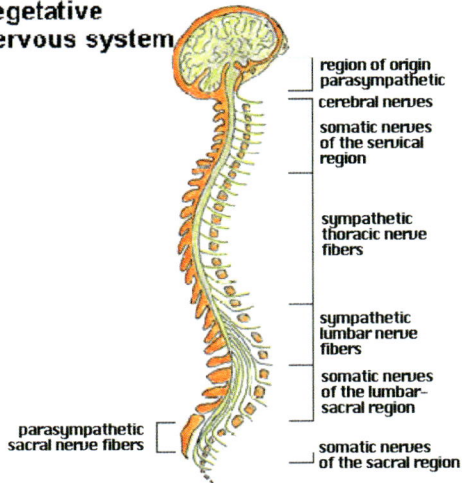

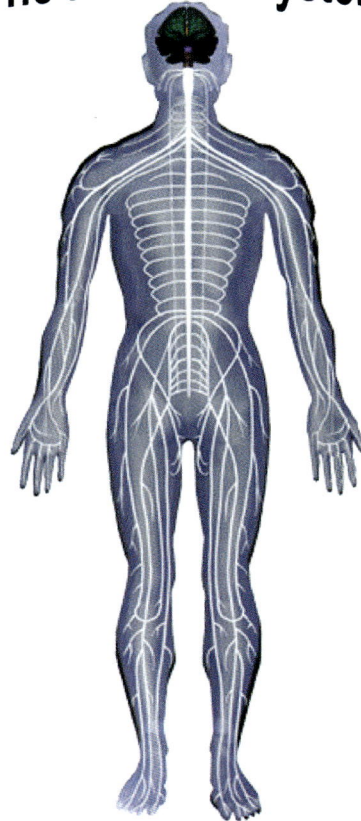

## The Nervous System

## The Brain

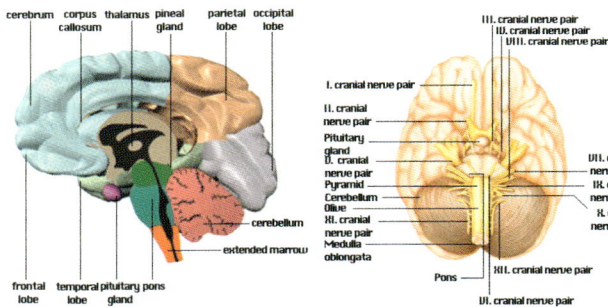

## The Ear

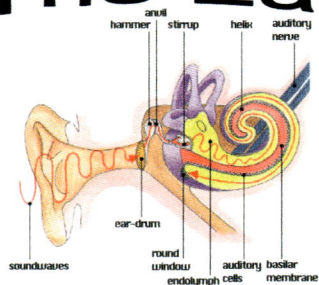

## The Eye

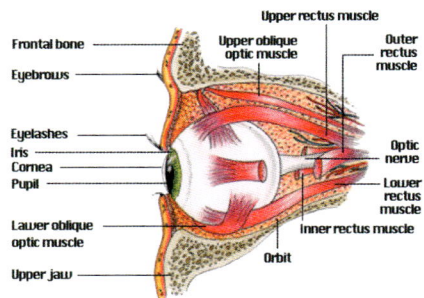

Body Illustrations from Human 3D, Mega Systems, Duluth, GA    www.mega-systems.net

comfort but because you will never be able to get the information from your **Higher Wisdom** on what to do next if you focus solely on the throbbing.

## Step 3: Letter "H" - Hear the Message

In the example of your cut finger, you will almost immediately know why you were cut. The message may be something obvious, like, "Yoo-hoo, it's not smart to stick your finger in the blender when it's moving." Or something more subliminal, like, "You know you shouldn't be cutting tomatoes with a dull knife while the kids are screaming and you're too tired."

Unfortunately, most of us simply tune out when it comes to serious illness by simply using the old standby: "I don't know why." However, as I mentioned earlier, stress comes in many forms, and emotional stress is the one that wreaks more havoc in the human body than any other. It's a silent presence that eats away at our cells, raises cortisol levels, knocks out our energy centers, and puts us smack into Dis- Ease.

In order to "hear the message" that is at the root of the illness, we must learn how to quiet the mind and listen to our Higher Wisdom. There is no other way that I know of to get the information. It doesn't show up on any x-ray or any other test for that matter. It lies hidden within our sub-conscious and must be drawn out for us to deal with. When we can get the answers from our Higher Wisdom, speaking directly through our individual organs, we will have the blueprint for our own healing. In that blueprint lays the light of hope that waits for us at the end of the dark tunnel we call disease.

## Step 4: Letter "E" - Evaluate your Illness

After befriending our illness and eliminating our pain, we find ourselves finally hearing the messages. Now what? Well, now it's time to do our second "E": Evaluate Your Illness. This is pretty simple. Once we immediately get our message from cutting our finger, the next thing we do is look at the size of the cut. Do we need a big Band-Aid, or a small one? Is the wound deep and needing to be stitched? That seems to be pretty straightforward but again, when it comes to serious illness, the choices can be endless. How serious is this sickness? Do I need a specialist, a surgeon, or a nutritionist? Should I change my diet, take some supplements, or do I need a prescription medication? All of these factors need to be answered by YOU— not your family, your friends, or anyone else. You can listen to their advice, but, ultimately, it is your body and your life, and you must take control if you want to be totally healed.

So how do we do this? Easy. Create a log of all the information you receive by filling out the Funsheet that corresponds with the visualization that you are doing. Those answers then can be placed in either or both of the following charts that I have created for you - The House of Well Being Chart and Goal Sheet.

*How to Heal Completely*

To use this chart effectively, under each heading first write the PROBLEM next to "P" first, then write possible SOLUTIONS next to "S" i.e. under Physical Health, next to P - Bring down brain swelling. Next to S – 1) Get an MRI 2) Ask Dr. for recommendati ns. 3) Take those suggestions into visualization #4 and ask your Higher Wisdom "Which is best for me?"

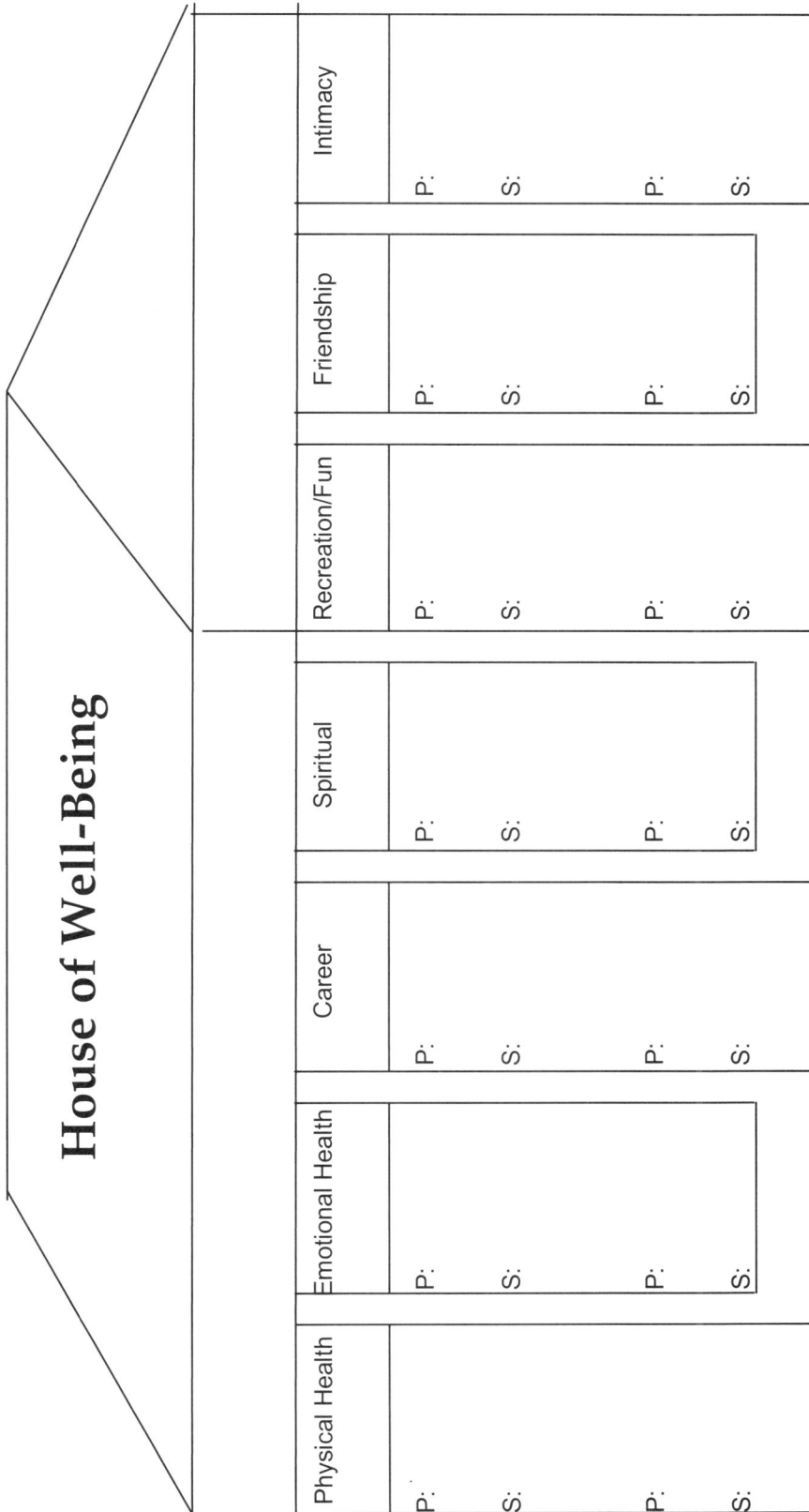

# House of Well-Being

| Physical Health | Emotional Health | Career | Spiritual | Recreation/Fun | Friendship | Intimacy |
|---|---|---|---|---|---|---|
| P: | P: | P: | P: | P: | P: | P: |
| S: | S: | S: | S: | S: | S: | S: |
| P: | P: | P: | P: | P: | P: | P: |
| S: | S: | S: | S: | S: | S: | S: |

The House of Well Being Chart was designed for you to look at all the aspects of you life. Under each heading write down the problems you have been experiencing next to the letter "P. " After you do your visualizations and start getting some answers, all you have to do is place the solutions you may have received under the letter "S," and you now have the beginnings of a simple "to do" list to follow.

As you complete and heal one problem at a time, simply check it off the chart. If you start developing more problems, create a new chart to get it handled quickly. What I've attempted to do is to place all your challenges on one 8 1/2" x 11" piece of paper, so that you can see the entire picture of your present situation at one glance. If you can see all the challenges of your life from this perspective, you won't get overwhelmed.

Under each leg, write down the challenges you are presently facing, if there are none in any particular leg, simply "x" that leg out. I suggest you do this first before we continue.

## Importance of Goals

The Goal Sheet was designed for you to get to the emotional and mental causes of your illnesses and other life challenges. It too is a road map to help you clear out those bodies. Dr. David D. Burns, in his book "Feeling Good," observed that the thought comes first, then the emotions. Science is now discovering that the body responds to our thoughts and emotions. In order to unravel the mystery of your illness, the logical steps would be to work backwards: starting from the illness, then back to the emotions that are causing it, then finally to the thoughts that created the emotions.

*Today's Date* _____    **Goal Sheet**    *Target Date* <u>ASASWA</u>

| Challenge | Desired Results | Mental Cause | Emotional Cause | Date Reached |
|---|---|---|---|---|
| Physical 1) | | | | |
| 2) | | | | |
| 3) | | | | |
| Career/Finance 1) | | | | |
| 2) | | | | |
| 3) | | | | |
| Relationship/ Recreation 1) | | | | |
| 2) | | | | |
| 3) | | | | |
| Spiritual/Other 1) | | | | |
| 2) | | | | |
| 3) | | | | |

Start by putting today's date in the left-hand corner of the Goal Sheet. As you can see, the Target Date on the right says "ASASWA." That stands for "As Soon As Spirit Will Allow." That declaration calls for the fastest solutions to the challenges you have listed. Please take a moment now to fill out the first column. Under Challenge, name the problems you wish to tackle under that heading. Then go across to column number four and write your best possible outcome under Desired Results. For example, under the heading Physical, write "Diabetes" or whatever illness is challenging you. Then under the column headed Desired Results, you may wish to write "to completely heal" or "to reduce my medication. " Choose whatever you think might be possible for you right now. If, for instance, you are not presently experiencing a specific illness and wrote under Physical, "Always tired," under Desired Results, you may wish to write something like "a healthier body" or "increase stamina" or "a stronger/firmer body" Or you may even try "a lighter body" if under Physical you wrote "lose weight". Gee, why didn't I think of that till now?

Under Career/Finance, you may wish to increase your income, pay off some debts, or find a job that you love. Please understand that you don't necessarily have to get a new job to increase your income. You simply have to ask Creator to send you some more prosperity. Such a request could get you a raise, a part-time situation, or have things happen in your world that would reduce your expenses so that you can stay at a job that you enjoy. On the other hand, if you absolutely hate your job, then by all means write "new career" or "new job" under Desired Results.

Under Relationship/Recreation you may wish to cite that you need more friends or someone to come forward with whom you can have a more intimate relationship. Under Spiritual you may wish to cite areas like "being able to feel more connected to God," or "being able to talk with my angels." These are just some examples.

You get the idea. The two middle columns, Emotional Cause and

Mental Cause, will be filled in when you get the answers in your visualizations, or feel free to fill it in immediately if you get an instant revelation while you are writing the question. What we are doing here is allowing you to see at a glance that what you have been thinking and feeling has brought you to the present situation. In order for you to get your desired results, you are going to have to make some changes in your thought processes. Before you can do that, you need to become aware of the thoughts that created the emotions that led to the challenge in the first place. You also need to be made aware that those thoughts and emotions are not in alignment with what you really want. In this way you can re-program your thinking with new phrases. The new phrases and thoughts will then create more positive emotions and together, they will support your Desired Results. Do I hear an "AH HA" coming?

It is important that you fill out both the House of Well Being Chart on page 27 and the Goal Sheet on page 29 before you start your visualizations. These will create the base line of what is going on now so that you know what questions to ask when you are called to do so in you visualizations. I suggest that you fill out both sheets now. You may choose to use the templates we've provided at the back of the book to copy them onto a larger piece of paper to make it easier for yourself and have a few extra handy.

## Step 5:  Letter "A" -  Absolve all four Bodies

We are now ready to start our letter "A": Absolve all your four bodies. Going back again to the cut finger analogy, you now know what size bandage you need, but first you MUST clean out the wound. You can use soap and water, peroxide or iodine. In the case of your internal physical body, you must detox. By that, I mean get rid of all the poisons, chemicals, heavy metals, and plaque build-up in your system. You may even have to flush out some of your major organs.

In the case of your mental body, you must be willing to stop the negative thoughts about your illness from creeping into your head and backing you into the "Fear" corner. The simple prayer, "Mind be still and know that I am love," will take care of that very nicely. Also, you must check every word you say. When you say, "my arthritis" or "my diabetes," you continually lay claim or own the illness and keep that negative energy going. Be very careful about what you say. We'll talk more about that later.

To absolve the spiritual body, all you need to do is pray or visualize daily and stay connected to your source. I would suggest that you honor your own personal spiritual beliefs and use them to help expand your awareness. Remember to keep an open mind and to allow the warm, loving, generous spirit of our Creator to be a part of your everyday life. That will keep you clear and able to move quickly into higher states of awareness. In the case of absolving your emotional body, you MUST clear out the big three: Guilt, Anger, and most of all, Fear. My angels have told me point blank that those three negative emotions are at the root of any and all illnesses. They said that if we are not willing to forgive others and ourselves for being human, if we are not willing to give up the guilt trips that we lay on ourselves and if we are not willing to walk through our fears, the emotional body will not let go. The energy that brought about the illness in the first place will still be intact, no matter how many pills or supplements we take, no matter how many treatments we go for, or how hard we diet.

I cannot emphasize this enough. Your illness was born in your negative thoughts, which created an upset in your emotional body and then moved into the physical body. You don't have to take my word for it. There have been many learned individuals and quantum physicists who have shared these similar thoughts. You can find them in film documentaries such as *What the Bleep do we Know* and my favorite *The Secret*. I'm giving you the opportunity to discover that for yourself. After a few visualizations, you will be able to find your own truth on the matter.

## Step 6: Letter "L" – Line up Physical Assistance

We have now absolved our four bodies and have made the notations on our Funsheets and on our charts, and so we now have the answers we need to do our "L," which is Line up Physical Assistance. Going back to the example of a cut finger, physical assistance is the ointment. It helps the wound heal by keeping bacteria out. If we translate the ointment to your illness, it would mean to get the advice of those people that you were internally guided to see. Then check their advice against your own internal meter before you move forward. Make sure that everyone is on the same page and that you are not being led to do something that goes against your grain.

If you feel uncomfortable taking the advice of any of these people, it may be that the lesson is one to overcome your own fear and to trust what you are getting, and not allow someone else to dictate what is right for you. Or it may be simply that you need to look further.

Another possibility could be that you are not ready to take their advice because the timing is wrong. In any case, I would suggest that you say a prayer of declaration; something like, "Creator, I am ready to receive the person or information that can best help me reach my healing goals." In that way, our Creator will provide you with all the assistance that you need.

Lining up physical assistance also includes acquiring the items that you may need to assist the body. Please notice that I said "acquire" and not "buy." Sometimes, your Creator will give you things through other people and you don't necessarily have to make a purchase. Have you ever considered the thought that something you need or desire may be gifted to you? My dental assistant once gave me the moulds that hold the bleaching gel without charging me $200, just because she wanted to reciprocate an act of kindness. That brings us to our next letter.

## Step 7:  Letter "E" -  Execute the Program

You now know what to do, so like Nike says, "Just do it. " Don't stand there and look at your finger bleeding, take care of it and keep changing the dressing until it's healed.  You will not only feel like a great burden has been lifted, but you will also feel a great sense of accomplishment and pride at being able to move your illness out quickly.  It's the greatest feeling in the world.  Well, let me rephrase that: almost the greatest feeling in the world.  Gee, I almost forgot about that.

## Step 8:  Letter "D" – Declare Thanks to Your Creator

That's like putting a Band-Aid on your finger.  When you absolutely know that you are protected, you can go forward.  If you can truly bless your illness and thank God for bringing it into your world, you've not only gotten your diploma; you've graduated with honors.  It means that you got it.  What did you get?  That you were simply sitting in the classroom called Sickness 101, which in truth is a life-altering friend that came into your world to enlighten you and to be your greatest teacher.  That is what illness truly is.

# Chapter 3

## Making the Letters Work for You

## Letter "B"

Let's go back to the beginning of our sequence of "How to Be Healed," starting with the Letter B. The best way I know how to befriend your illness is to first learn how to relax. So I came up with this exercise to help you tune into your body more closely, and to become familiar with your personal energy flow and how that effects movement in your body.

Take a look at Funsheet #1: Opening to Heal on the following page. Grab a pen and write today's date at the top. In this way you will be creating a diary or a log of your progress. These sheets were designed to help you become aware of the growth of your own intuition by recording your sessions.

As you can see, I've numbered your intuitive levels from zero to three. At level zero: You have no feeling or awareness whatsoever. At level one: You may experience a mild sensation, but really can't make it out. At level two: You may feel a medium sensation and may even have a clue as to what it means. At level three: You may experience a strong sensation and be able to identify the feeling—like hot, cold, agitated, sad, disappointed, happy.

This exercise has two parts. First we're going to focus on a particular area of your body, and then you are going to put a circle around the number that corresponds with your level of awareness of that body part in the "before" column. You may also want to jot down a note or two right next to the name of the corresponding chakra. Are you ready?

Today's Date _____

# Funsheet #1

## Visualization #1 – Opening to Heal

**Intuitive Levels** 0 - None

1 - Feel mild sensation/presence but cannot identify

2 - Feel a medium sensation and some identification

3 - Feel a strong sensation and able to identify easily

| Locations of Intuitive Centers | Intuitive Level | |
|---|---|---|
| | *Before* | *After* |
| 1) Root_____ | 0 - 1 - 2 - 3 | 0 - 1 - 2 - 3 |
| 2) Pelvis _____ | 0 - 1 - 2 - 3 | 0 - 1 - 2 - 3 |
| 3) Solar Plexus _____ | 0 - 1 - 2 - 3 | 0 - 1 - 2 - 3 |
| 4) Heart _____ | 0 - 1 - 2 - 3 | 0 - 1 - 2 - 3 |
| 5) Throat _____ | 0 - 1 - 2 - 3 | 0 - 1 - 2 - 3 |
| 6) Brow _____ | 0 - 1 - 2 - 3 | 0 - 1 - 2 - 3 |
| 7) Crown _____ | 0 - 1 - 2 - 3 | 0 - 1 - 2 - 3 |

**Comments:**

_____

_____

I'd like you to close your eyes and take a long, deep breath. Hold it for the count of 7 then exhale. With your eyes still closed, focus on your root chakra. It is located at the end of your tailbone and wraps around your frontal region. Stay focused for 10 seconds, then open your eyes. What did you feel—anything? Choose a number in the "before" column that corresponds with your experience and circle it.

Now, close your eyes again. Inhale slowly and deeply, and hold the breath for the count of 7. Exhale. This time, focus your attention on your pelvic area across your abdomen. Again try to stay focused for 10 full seconds, then open your eyes and jot down what you are experiencing there. Choose a number, and then close your eyes again.

Inhale; hold the breath for 7. Exhale. Focus your attention on your solar plexus, which is above your belly button at mid-stomach. Do you feel anything there? Now, open your eyes and choose a number, then close your eyes again.

Inhale; hold the breath for 7. Exhale. Pay attention to your heart. Is it beating normally, or is something else going on? Stay there for 10 seconds. Open your eyes and make your notations, then close your eyes again.

Inhale; hold the breath for 7. Exhale. Focus on your throat for 10. Open your eyes and pick a number, then close your eyes once more.

Inhale; hold the breath for 7. Exhale and focus on the center of your brow. Any tension there? Check for 10. Now open your eyes and mark your sheet and close your eyes one last time.

Inhale; hold the breath for 7. Exhale. Then focus on the top of your head for 10. Open your eyes and make your final notations.

Now that we have an idea of where your intuition levels are, we have what the doctors call a base line. It's the first measuring point from which you can go either up or down. Of course, I know that you're only going up. That's what this is all about: getting to know yourself better.

## Four States of Consciousness

Before you get ready for your first visualization, I would like to explain the four states of consciousness that we go through during the course of the day. We start by being fully awake and we end with falling sound asleep. When we are fully awake, walking, talking, listening and responding, we are in what is called the Beta state. In that state the brain is moving at over 16 EEGs, or electroencephalographic waves, per second. Sounds real technical, doesn't it? EEG is a whole lot easier to remember. As we quiet down, our brains go to the next stage of consciousness, which is called Alpha. In the Alpha state, our brain waves are operating at about 12-14 EEGs per second. This is also called the Meditative State. Then, as we get more relaxed, we go through Theta, which is about 8-10 EEGs per second, and finally, we land into Delta, or REM sleep, which is our unconscious sleep stage. In Delta, our brain is operating at about 4-6 EEGs and we are completely asleep. So the four stages of consciousness again are: Beta, Alpha, Theta and Delta.

You might say that Alpha is the normal first phase of our sleep process. It is there that we can do our best work, and it is in that state that we can receive the answers we're looking for. If you do fall asleep, not to worry—my guides and teachers assure me that you will still receive the information you need on a subliminal level. Sometimes we simply need to get out of the way to allow the healing to begin. When you are ready to receive the information on a conscious level, you will have no trouble staying awake.

## Preparing to Visualize

It's time for you to get ready for your first visualization. I suggest that you sit in a comfortable chair or be slightly reclined. If you prefer to lie down, then keep your knees bent, with your feet on the floor, or the mattress and your head elevated on a pillow or two, so that you don't fall asleep. It's important for you to remain awake and stay in Alpha, and not to fall into Theta or Delta. Pop Visualization #1 *Opening to Heal* into your player if you have one, or read the following text into your personal recorder first, then relax as you play it back and listen to your own voice. You may choose to have your favorite meditative music playing in the background as you record.

When you see instructions in italics, please follow them. They are placed here for you to get the best possible experience. When you see *(pause)* in the script, allow yourself between 4-6 seconds before reading/recording the next sentence. Some of the directions may call for more time, i.e. 15, 30 or 60 seconds. These longer pauses are placed to give you enough time to see clearly or to hear the messages that are being presented to you.

## Visualization #1- *Opening to Heal*

Get into a very comfortable position. Place the tips of your thumb and index fingers of each hand together to form a circle and make the okay sign. Keeping your fingers in the okay position, turn your hands palms up. Now rest them either on top or along side your legs. Now close your eyes. Begin to drift with the music as it gently flows over you.

Imagine a large blackboard in front of you. Inhale deeply. Hold the breath *(for the count of 7)*. Exhale slowly. See the numbers 3, 3, 3. Inhale. Hold the breath (for the count of 7). Exhale. See the numbers 2, 2, 2. Inhale. Hold the breath *(for the count of 7)*. Exhale. See the numbers 1, 1, 1.

Focus your attention on your head and face. "I thank you for the ability to think - see-smell-hear and for the ability to feel soothing breezes on my face. I thank you for the wonder of my communication skills, my thought process and creative ideas. See your head in a beautiful pink spotlight. Cover it completely in this soft pink light. You'll feel a tingling sensation, a feeling of warmth. This part of your body is now calm, rested and serene.

Focus your attention on your throat, shoulders, and upper chest area. "I thank you for my ability to speak, for upholding my principles and for meeting the challenges of this life. I thank you for the ability to express my creativity and accept my nourishment. " Cover your throat, shoulders and upper chest area with the soft pink light… You'll feel a tingling sensation, a feeling of warmth. This part of your body is now calm, rested and serene.

Focus your attention on your arms and hands…"I thank you for the ability to feel and hold the pleasures of this life, for my balance and for lifting me to higher places. I thank you for warning me of danger and for helping to protect me." Cover your arms and hands with the soft pink light. You'll feel and tingling sensation, a feeling of warmth. This part of your body is calm, rested and serene.

Focus your attention on your heart, lungs and abdomen. "I thank you for the feelings of joy, love, happiness and all my emotions. I thank you for my ease of breathing. I especially thank you for nourishing me and for giving me energy and the power of movement." Now cover your heart, lungs and abdomen with a soft pink light. You'll feel a tingling sensation, a feeling of warmth. This part of your body is now calm, rested and serene.

Focus your attention on your lower abdomen and pelvic area. "I thank you for cleansing me and eliminating poisons from my body and for bringing forth new life and creativity." Cover your lower abdomen and pelvic area with a soft pink light. You'll feel a tingling sensation, a feeling of warmth. Now this part of your body is calm, rested and serene.

Focus your attention of your right leg, from hip to ankle. "I thank you for moving me forward and taking me through the first steps of this life. I thank you for your grace and flexibility and for carrying me from place to place and supporting my body." Cover your entire right leg with a soft pink light. You'll feel a tingling sensation, a feeling of warmth. This part of your body is now calm, rested and serene.

Focus your attention on your left leg, from hip to ankle. "I thank you for moving me forward from one goal to another and for taking great strides in this life experience. I thank you for helping me to distribute my weight evenly and carrying me in all directions." Cover your left leg with a soft pink light. You'll feel a tingling sensation, a feeling of warmth. This part of your body is now calm, rested and serene.

Focus your attention on your feet. "I thank you for stabilizing my body and grounding me. I thank you for the pleasure of running, jumping, kicking and dancing and for my freedom of mobility. I thank you for allowing all negative energy to escape through the soles and for your continual support." Cover your feet in a soft pink light. You'll feel a tingling sensation, a feeling of warmth. This part of your body is now calm, rested and serene.

Focus your attention on your hands. Turn your hands palms up. Place your thumb and index fingers of each hand together forming a circle as if you were going to pinch something. Say this to yourself after me. "Whenever I put these two fingers of either hand together in this manner, my mind automatically reaches this level of consciousness to balance and heal my body, neutralize pain and reach my higher understanding."

Now visualize a beautiful silver white light coming down from above you to surround your soft pink light. It is now forming a large silver white pyramid around your entire body. Say this to yourself after me. "Beloved Creator, I ask for the white light of protection, over me, under me, around and about, in and out and in all the nooks and crannies. I ask that my DNA light filaments be re-connected that I may be awakened to my highest understanding. I ask that my brow chakra be opened so I may see that which goes beyond the physical realm and I ask that my crown chakra be opened to receive your wisdom. So be it. So it is. "

Now focus your attention on the base of your spine. See the golden light of strength covering your tailbone and say to yourself, "I command from the love essence of my being that my root chakra, my center of creativity be balanced, whole and complete. So be it. So it is." Inhale and pull up the golden light to your pelvis. Exhale.

"I command from the love essence of my being that my pelvic chakra, my center of serenity, be balanced, whole and complete. So be it. So it is." (Inhale and pull up the golden light to mid stomach. Exhale.)

"I command from the love essence of my being that my solar plexus chakra, my center of intuitive feeling, be balanced whole and complete. So be it. So it is." Inhale and pull up the golden light to your heart. Exhale.

"I command from the love essence of my being that my heart chakra, my center of love, be balanced, whole and complete. So be it. So it is." Inhale and pull up the golden light to your throat. Exhale.

"I command from the love essence of my being that my throat chakra, my center of communication, be balanced, whole and complete. So be it. So it is." Inhale and pull up the golden light to the center of your brow, your third eye and exhale.

"I command from the love essence of my being that my brow chakra, my ability to see that which is unseen, be balanced, whole and complete. So be it. So it is." Inhale and pull up the golden light to the top of your head and exhale.

"I command from the love essence of my being that my crown chakra, my center of spirituality and connection to Creator, be balanced, whole and complete. So be it. So it is. "

Focus your attention on the top of your head. See a bright emerald green light enter the top of your head and fill your entire body with a pleasant crisp, clean sensation. Allow the light to travel to all parts of your body and exit all negativity through the soles of your feet. Inhale and drink in green light and say to yourself, "I change my reality and accept my blessings now. I am healed…I am peace…I am healed…I am joy…I am healed…I am longevity of life…I am healed…I am love…I am healed…I am harmony…I am healed…I am balance…I am healed…Health I am…Health I am…Health I am… So be it and so it is. "

Count from one to five. At each number you will become more and more alert. One - beginning to come up now, two - becoming more alert, three - halfway there, four - almost home, five - open your eyes fully awake and feeling great.

## Funsheet #1 Notations

Congratulations, you've just taken the first step into raising your awareness. I promise you the journey only gets better. That should have been pretty easy. Pick up Funsheet #1 again. This time, I suggest that you write some notes about your experiences during your visualization in the "comments" portion at the bottom of the page. Write down anything of importance, like: "I felt tingles," or "I felt lighter, calmer," or maybe you saw something or heard something—anything that occurred that is even slightly different than your normal state of consciousness.

After you've finished with your comments, close your eyes and go through your chakras once more taking in a deep breath, holding for the count of 7, exhaling, then focusing on the chakra you're working on. This time, remember what happened to them in the visualization and how they may have changed. Make your evaluations for each by choosing the numbers under the column marked "After."

# Chapter 4

## Eliminating Pain / Negativity / Fever

## Letter "E"

Let's keep moving down our list to our next letter "E," as in Eliminate Pain. As I said before, you cannot get to the next letter until you are able to get the pain under control. In our next visualization we will be doing two different things at the same time: first, focusing away from the pain, and secondly, adding the energy of color to get our best results.

In the last visualization, you balanced your chakras by using prayers of action. By saying, "I command from the Love essence of my being," you sent forth words of intent. Since you and Creator are a team, your chakras got the message to balance out.

In our next visualization, we're going to do something different. We're going to balance the chakras with shape and color. Now take a look at the Chakra Symbol Chart on page 20.

As you can see each chakra not only has its own symbol, but it also has a primary color and a balancing color. Individual charkas can also be balanced by playing, singing or toning its designated or harmonic note.

Our root chakra is represented by a square, and it is typically the color of red, which is appropriate since it is the seat of our passion. It is passion that allows us to create everything in our world, from a new career to a beautiful poem. The harmonizing, or balancing, color for the root is a bright Kelly green, and its harmonious note is "C," as in doe: "Doe, a dear…" Whoops I'm slipping into Maria.

Our next chakra is the pelvic chakra. I call it the center of serenity, because when it's out of balance, we're usually nervous, agitated, and off kilter. The pelvic chakra is symbolized by an orange, inverted triangle, and can be balanced with a more yellowish orange. Its harmonious note is "E."

Now, moving along, we have the solar plexus chakra, which many call our second brain. It is the gut-feeling center, and it always warns us of trouble. Its symbol is the quarter moon and its color is yellow. It can be balanced by using the color off-white, and its harmonious note is "D."

The heart chakra is probably the easiest to recognize. We often feel its flutter when we look at someone we love, but we can also hear it pounding the instant we suspect that we might be in danger. What most of us fail to recognize is that every time we have a negative thought about our life circumstances, like, "Am I ever going to get that promotion? " or, "Is he ever going to love me? " or, "I'm so worried about so and so," we create a stress signal or a light thump. Because this thump or electrical impulse goes unnoticed, we don't think we're doing ourselves any harm, but if we keep thinking those negative thoughts all day long, we put ourselves through constant stress. It should come as no surprise that heart disease is the number one killer in the United States today. The heart chakra is represented by the hexagon, and its color is grass green. Its balancing color is violet, and its harmonic note is "F."

Our throat chakra not only controls our speaking voice, but it also controls our nose, our sinuses, and our eyes. When we're having any type of upper respiratory infection or problem, the throat is out of balance. Since it represents communication, it is also the center of telepathy with Creator, the angels and everyone on the other side. Its symbol is two concentric circles, which are turquoise, its balancing color is sky blue and its harmonizing note is "G."

Our brow chakra is commonly referred to as our third eye. It rests above our pituitary gland and it is our center of inner vision. When it is blocked, we have difficulty envisioning our future, or solutions to even simple challenges. You might say that we are blinded by our own ignorance or unwillingness to expand our world. Its symbol is a blue dot and its balancing color is pink. It can also be balanced by toning the note "A."

And lastly, our crown chakra is located above our head. It is not only our center of spirituality, but it is the point where we, or our consciousness, enters and exits the body everyday. Think of it as a dimmer switch. At night when we go to sleep, our brain waves slow down and we slowly slip out of the crown chakra leaving just enough juice behind to keep the bodily functions purring. That's why we feel cold and reach for a blanket because we've let some energy out of the body so that it can rest. When we come back in the morning, we open our eyes and gradually get back into Beta or maybe not. Have you ever felt like you crash-landed and woke up suddenly? That's just your consciousness hurrying back. The symbol for the crown chakra is the Star of David. Its color is magenta, which is sort of a purplish-red, and its harmonizing note is "B."

When one or more of your chakras are out of balance, you are either in pain, stressed out, or sick. Let's start with pain. Why do you suppose pain comes about? Well, here again, the doctors will tell us that pain is the body's protective signal. It's a way of calling our attention to a problem in the workings of the body. However pain, too, takes on many faces. It can be physical pain, like when we get stung by a bee or break a leg, or it can be emotional pain, like when we continually cry over a loss in our life. Then, of course, there is mental pain—the kind that keeps us up till all hours of the night with worry. All of this pain eventually settles into the physical body and starts doing some type of damage.

In my experience, the pain will show up in the part of your body that is most susceptible to your root issue. For instance, if your mental body is worried about finances or support issues, your back might go out because your spine supports your entire body. If your emotional body is reeling from a relationship issue, that could easily land in a digestion or an elimination problem. If your mental body is worried "out of its mind," those types of issues could wreak havoc on your heart or give you an ulcer.

Truthfully, your emotional and mental issues could show up anywhere, depending on your personality, your belief system and what priorities you hold dear. It would be impossible for me, or anyone, to venture a guess as to where your underlying cause will manifest in the body. We are all uniquely individual. I've had money issues show up in my sinuses and my throat where I would normally suspect communication issues. That's why I wrote visualizations number three and number four, so you could get to the issue that brought about your present illness. You see most of us are unaware of the underlying circumstances of our life and without that information and a plan to resolve those issues, it could take you years to clear out the negativity and to heal.

Take your time with this next visualization. It is very important to developing a strong mind/body connection. Even if you are not presently experiencing any pain, at present this visualization will clear out any negativity which can potentially harm you. Most importantly, this visualization will also help you learn to focus on a single object. When you master focusing, you gain control over pain. Eventually you gain control over your body and your life. That's when I believe you can heal anything.

**Today's Date** _____

# Funsheet #2

## Meditation #2 – Eliminating/Pain/Negativity/Fever

**Pain/Negativity Levels**
0 - Completely calm/relaxed/pain free
1 - Feeling tense/tired/slightly uncomfortable
2 - Some agitation/nervousness/noticeable
  discomfort
3 - In stress/pain apparent
4 - Agitated/throbbing pain
5 - Highly agitated/unbearable pain

**Locations of Discomfort/Stress**      **Pain/Negativity Level**

|  | *Before* | *After* |
|---|---|---|
| 1) _____ | 0 - 1 - 2 - 3 - 4 – 5 | 0 - 1 - 2 - 3 - 4 –5 |
| 2) _____ | 0 - 1 - 2 - 3 - 4 - 5 | 0 - 1 - 2 - 3 - 4 - 5 |
| 3) _____ | 0 - 1 - 2 - 3 - 4 - 5 | 0 - 1 - 2 - 3 - 4 - 5 |
| 4) _____ | 0 - 1 - 2 - 3 - 4 – 5 | 0 - 1 - 2 - 3 - 4 - 5 |
| 5) _____ | 0 - 1 - 2 - 3 - 4 - 5 | 0 - 1 - 2 - 3 - 4 - 5 |

**Comments:**

_____

_____

_____

As you can see in Funsheet #2 – Eliminating Pain/Negativity/ Fever, I have added two more levels. Jot down today's date at the top. As you can see, pain level zero is pain free. That's what we're aiming for by the end of the visualization, but any movement down is good your first time out. Most of my students are able to drop two levels very quickly.

Level one is only slightly uncomfortable. Level two is noticeable discomfort. Level three is high stress and pain. Level four is throbbing, and level five is unbearable. Decide which areas of the body you would like to work on and write them in under the heading "LOCATIONS OF DISCOMFORT AND STRESS. " I've given you up to five spaces to fill in but I suggest that you start with one or two. You can try more when you're able to focus clearly and get information easily. Next to each body part, measure your pain level by choosing one level from the chart and circling it in the "Before" column, just as you did with the last Funsheet.

Next to number one under the column "Locations of Discomfort and Stress," you can write, say, "left thumb. " Now, since your thumb is throbbing from a recent wound, you would circle the number four under the "Before" column. You get the idea. Take a minute now and choose the parts that you will be working on, then evaluate

Now that we know what we're working on, I'd like to give you a few pointers on how to get the most out of this visualization. Eliminating pain takes practice. You may have to do this visualization several times before you can get your desired results. Just don't give up. As I said before, this is a skill-building program. The more you practice, the better you'll get. Remember, even experienced meditators usually need a good twenty minutes to stop pain and it may take them two tries before they can get the pain down to zero. So please don't get discouraged. Dropping your pain level even one notch is a triumph because you did it by yourself without the help of any drugs.

If you're running a fever, try this visualization in a bathtub of warm water. Now please be careful about electrical wires in the bathroom near the tub. Neither one of us needs to hear our favorite news anchor say, "Student electrocuted while attempting to heal in the bathtub, film at eleven "

After you finish your visualization, go back to Funsheet #2, circle your "After" pain levels and fill in your comments. Take note of anything that came to your attention during the visualization. This will help you immensely and remind you what to look for the next time you do the visualization.

Let's get comfortable. Pop in Visualization #2: *Eliminating Pain / Negativity / Fever* or record the following script into your cassette deck. Please note that the first few minutes are almost identical to Visualization #1 and will be so on Visualizations #3 and #4 as well. It's not a mistake. The best way to achieve an alpha state is to repeat the same sequence over and over until you memorize it and can do it without any help. Then you can play for favorite music piece and go for it solo.

## Visualization #2 - *Eliminating Pain/Fever/Negativity*

Get into a very comfortable position. Place the tips of your thumb and index fingers of each hand together to form a circle and make the okay sign. Keeping your fingers in the okay position, turn your hands palms up. Now rest them either on top or along side your legs. Close your eyes. Begin to drift with the music as it gently flows over you.

Imagine a large blackboard in front of you. Inhale deeply. Hold the breath *(for the count of 7)*. Exhale slowly. See the numbers 3, 3, 3. Inhale. Hold the breath *(for the count of 7)*. Exhale. See the numbers 2, 2, 2. Inhale. Hold the breath *(for the count of 7)*. Exhale. See the numbers 1, 1, 1.

Focus your attention on your hands. Turn your hands palms up. Place your thumb and index finger of each hand together to form a circle as if you were going to pinch something. Now say this to yourself after me "Whenever I put these two fingers of either hand together in this manner, my mind automatically reaches this level of consciousness to balance and heal my body, neutralize pain and reach my higher understanding.

Focus your attention on the area that is giving you pain or difficulty. Tell this body part how much you love it and thank it for all the work that it does for you. *(pause)* Apologize for any action on your part that may have caused it to become distressed. Tell it that you wish to make peace. *(pause)* Tell it that you are going to help it release all the negative energy surrounding it so that it can come back to perfect balance. *(pause)*

Now say, "I command from the Love Essence of My Being that all the negative energy creating this pain leave my body now. *(pause)* I am thankful for the opportunity to overcome this challenge and release all this pain back to the universe with love."

Now visualize red smoke rising out of the painful area. Push it out. Push it out. Watch the smoke rise and start to form a tiny fiery red ball about the size of a small pea. It is floating about two feet in front of you. *(pause)* Now say, "I command from the Love Essence of My Being that this negative energy go into the ball." *(pause)* Keep pushing it out. Watch the tiny fireball. It is getting hotter and hotter, brighter and brighter, larger and larger, and more and more intense.

As the ball keeps growing, it pulls all your pain into the center. Watch it grow. It gathers all the pain and is now the size of a marble. It swirls around and around collecting even more red smoke. It is getting hotter and hotter, brighter and brighter, larger and larger, and more and more intense.

You can actually feel the heat in front of you as your fireball grows to the size of a candy gumball. It is spinning much faster now, collecting negative energy as it continues to grow hotter and hotter, brighter and brighter, larger and larger, and more and more intense.

Stay focused on your fireball.  Watch it take on even more red smoke. It has now grown to the size of a ping-pong ball.  *(pause)*  It is still small but growing hotter and hotter, brighter and brighter, larger and larger, and more and more intense.

Watch it gather more negative energy.  It spins like a top and gains more speed.  It has now grown to the size of a golf ball, still gathering smoke, still getting larger, growing hotter and hotter, brighter and brighter, larger and larger, and more and more intense.

See the red smoke swirling around and around.  *(pause)*  All the pain, the anger, the frustration, and guilt that you have been carrying is being caught up into this whirling ball.  *(pause)*  It has now grown to the size of a tennis ball and it's still getting hotter and hotter, brighter and brighter, larger and larger, and more and more intense.

Push the red smoke into your fireball.  Watch it spin like a ball of yarn. It moves.  It grows.  It is now the size of a baseball.  *(pause)*  It keeps getting hotter and hotter, brighter and brighter, larger and larger and more and more intense.

Keep pushing the negativity into your fireball.  *(pause)*  It's like a bottomless pit. *(pause)*  It can hold all that you can push into it.  So much so, that it has grown to the size of a softball, becoming hotter and hotter, brighter and brighter, larger and larger and more and more intense.  *(pause)*

The heat in front of you feels like a hot summer afternoon in the sun. Your fireball continues to grow.  It seems to feed on all your negative energy, encapsulating it to the size of a bocce ball.  Watch it become hotter and hotter, brighter and brighter, larger and larger and more and more intense.  *(pause)*

Look at its intensity.  Your fireball keeps growing and pulling all your pain right into its center. *(pause)* It's almost the size of volleyball now, getting hotter and hotter, brighter and brighter, larger and larger, and more and more intense. *(pause)*

Pay close attention to the swirling mass. It collects more and more negative energy and begins to take on a life of its own. It's now about the size of a soccer ball, growing hotter and hotter, brighter and brighter, larger and larger, and more and more intense. *(pause)*

The heat in front of you is getting stronger. *(pause)* Push all the negativity into the fireball with all your might. Come on now - push. See the ball expand to the size of a basketball. It's spinning hotter and hotter, brighter and brighter, larger and larger, and more and more intense. *(pause)*

Your fireball has become so strong; it takes on even more speed. The stream of red smoke has finally come to an end. The ball has collected all your negativity and all your pain. The outer layer of your fireball starts to cool down and seal its contents. For some strange reason it now begins to change its shape and looks very much like a football. Although it's still red, it is only warm to the touch. You have no problem handling it or touching it.

Now take the fiery red football into your strongest hand. Pull back and throw it as hard as you can towards the goal post far ahead in front of you. Watch it soar, 100 ft…200 ft…300 ft…400 ft…500 ft. and see it crest right over the center of the goal post and burst into tiny violet particles of light, just like a 4th of July skyrocket. Watch it as it fades into the night sky. It's gone now. It can no longer hurt you. *(pause)*

Come back to the body area that you have just cleansed. Visualize a blue-violet light covering the entire area and say, "I call forth the blue light of healing from the Love Essence of my being, to soothe, calm and re-balance my entire body". Now bring that blue-violet across your body and repeat after me. "I am cooled. I am healed. I am soothed. I am healed. I am relaxed. I am healed. I am balanced. I am healed. I am whole. I am healed."

Once again focus your attention on the base of your spine, your root chakra. See a beautiful red square floating over your tailbone. *(pause)* Now change the color of the square into a bright kelly green. *(pause)* Take a deep breath… and exhale.

Focus your attention on your abdomen, your pelvic chakra. Visualize a beautiful orange inverted triangle. Now change the color of your upside down triangle to more of a yellow orange. *(pause)* Take a deep breath…and exhale.

Focus your attention on your mid stomach, your solar plexus chakra. Visualize a yellow quarter moon. *(pause)* Now change the color of your crescent moon to off white. *(pause)* Take a deep breath…and exhale.

Focus your attention on your heart chakra. Visualize a grass green colored hexagon floating above your heart. *(pause)* Now change the color of your hexagon to violet. *(pause)* Take a deep breath…and exhale.

Focus your attention on your throat chakra. Visualize a small turquoise circle inside a larger turquoise circle. It is floating above your throat. *(pause)* Now change the colors of the circles to sky blue. *(pause)* Take a deep breath…and exhale.

Focus your attention on your brow chakra. Visualize a navy blue dot the size of a penny, floating above the center of your brow. *(pause)* Now change the color of your dot to light pink. *(pause)* Take a deep breath…and exhale.

Focus your attention on the top of your head, your crown chakra. Visualize a magnificent six-pointed star the color of magenta red floating above your head. *(pause)* Now change the color of the star to a bright gold. *(pause)* Take a deep breath and exhale. My entire body is now balanced, whole and complete. *(pause)*

It is now time for you to return to your outer reality. At the count of five, you will awaken completely rested and pain free. One - beginning to come up now, two - becoming more alert, three - halfway there, four - almost home, five - open your eyes fully awake and feeling great.

## Reminder - Take notes

I hope you thoroughly enjoyed your last visualization and are feeling somewhat better. Did you remember to fill in your Funsheet with your "after" evaluations? If not, take the time to do so now. Put in as much details as you can remember. Even the slightest feeling or smell can make a huge difference in how you move forward.

# Chapter 5

## Talking with Your Body

## Letter "H"

Before we can start working on our next letter, "H," to hear our messages, I thought it might be a good idea to get more familiar with your body parts. In that way, it will be easier for you to see where the messages are coming from. The most important discovery that I made during my healing challenges was that my body parts seem to have a mind and opinion of their own—totally different from mine. Go figure.

To get the most out of any healing program, I believe it's important to have at least a basic working knowledge of our bodies. Check out the illustrations on pages 21-24 to help you better visualize and understand the workings of the human body.

Let's start from the outside and work inside. Over a million cells come together to form our largest and most elastic organ that we call our skin. The skin's job is to protect our bodies from outside substances, while holding in vital water and salt levels. It also is responsible for our senses of touch and temperature. In some places it can be very thick, as in the soles of the feet, and in other places, it can be very thin, as in our eyelids. Our skin changes form according to its function. For instance, the skin around our elbows is loose so that we can bend, while the skin in the palm of our hand is taut, so that we can easily grip onto something. Every month we shed our old skin, and the new, underlying cells develop a whole new outer layer. If it's always brand new, then why, as we get older, is it coming in wrinkled? Is it because we look in the mirror, see a line, and accept that we're growing older, so that the next day, when a new cell is born, it corrupts into the same degenerative pattern? I wonder.

Our skin is also made up of several layers. The outside is called the epidermis. It is a layer of flat, dead cells that contain keratin, which makes the skin tough and waterproof. As the new cells move toward the surface, they harden. Some cells produce melanin, which darkens or pigments the outer layer and protects it from sunlight. Under the epidermis is a more elastic and thicker layer called the dermis. It contains nerve endings, blood vessels, elastic fibers, sweat glands that cool the skin, and glands that produce oil to keep our hair and skin supple. Beneath the dermis layer rests another layer called the hypodermis, which holds our fat, our blood vessels and our hair follicles.

Under our skin lies a layer of six hundred-fifty muscles. The ones we can control, like when you bend your knee or your finger is called voluntary muscles. They work in pairs, and are attached to our bones with elastic bands called tendons. When one muscle contracts, the other relaxes. That's how we create movement.

The other class of muscles is called the involuntary muscles. They work automatically, like our heart, our circulatory system and our digestive system. These muscles have their own rhythm and they move as needed.

Let's take a look at our skeleton. It lies beneath our muscles to support and protect our entire body. The front is made up of the skull, face bones, collarbones, breastbone and the ribs, which create a cage to protect our heart and lungs. Each bone is made up of three layers, housing living cells, nerves and blood vessels. The outside layer is thin and tough and is called the periosteum. It covers a strong layer, which in turn covers a sponge-like core. The cells of the periosteum can replace and repair broken bone. The hard layers underneath contain calcium, phosphorus and collagen. The inner, spongy layer is lightweight and looks like a honeycomb. The long bones in our arms and our legs, as well as our breastbone, contain a jelly-like substance called marrow in their central cavity. That is where our blood cells are made. In just one day, bone marrow can produce as many as five BILLION red blood cells. Amazing.

Although any one bone cannot bend, if we link them together, we can create movement. Our bones meet at the joints, which are held in place by bands. These are called "ligaments. " There are several type of joints. Our hip and shoulder joints look like a ball and socket. That allows for full rotation, while our finger joints are simple hinges that only allow for bending and straightening. Our wrist joint is called a pivot joint, which twists and turns. The movement of our joints is assisted by a smooth, "hyline" cartilage that covers the ends of the bones, and a thin sac or membrane containing "synovial" fluid. It is the synovial membrane that provides lubrication and prevents our bones from grinding together. Oftentimes, when our bones don't get the proper nourishment or move out of alignment, they begin to brush up against one another. The sac is broken and the bones begin to wear down. This is commonly called arthritis.

When we look at the spine we should view it from its two main functions. First, it protects the spinal cord, and secondly, it provides the supporting backbone of our entire skeleton. It contains twenty-four bones known as "vertebrae," starting at the base of the skull and ending with the "sacrum," which is shaped like a triangle. That is followed by the "coccyx," which is commonly called our tailbone. In between the vertebrae are small pillows called discs that are made up of a Jell-O-like substance. These discs, or pillows, between the vertebrae allow the spine to bend and twist. During the course of the day, we actually shrink because our discs become a little squashed. This makes us a little shorter than when we first got out of bed in the morning.

Now, let's take a look at our lungs.  The job of the lungs is to supply oxygen.  Without oxygen, our cells would die and we could not break down our food into the necessary energy, water, and carbon dioxide gas.  When we breathe out, the lungs push out the carbon dioxide and water.  This is called respiration.   The air is inhaled through our nose and mouth into the "trachea," or windpipe.  Then the air passes through two narrow tubes, called the "bronchi," where it is pulled into the lungs.  Inside each lung, there is a group of small branches that look like trees.  They are called the "bronchioles." The bronchioles end in tiny chambers called "alveoli," which are surrounded by tiny blood vessels.  The gasses cross the alveoli walls into the blood vessels, where they are picked up and carried to our various body parts.

Our breathing, however, is controlled by a muscle called the "diaphragm." When you inhale, your chest and ribs move out, and your diaphragm contracts and moves down.  When you exhale, your chest moves in and your diaphragm moves up.  This forces the air out of the lungs.  If your diaphragm contracts too quickly when you inhale, you are likely to get the hiccups.

That reminds me of a great remedy that was taught to me by my seventh-grade teacher, Mrs. Halpern.  When you get the hiccups, fill a wide mouth glass or cup with water.  Go over to a sink.  Bend over and pull your chin close to your chest.  Place your lips onto the opposite or the "wrong" side of the glass.  Tilt the bottom of the glass toward the underside of your chin and drink upside down.  Depending on the width of the glass, you chin may well fit inside the opening.  In that position, you force the air out of the diaphragm and the hiccups stop immediately.  It works for me every time.

When we view our blood and circulatory system, we see that it is made up of four components: red blood cells, white blood cells, platelets, and liquid plasma.  Not only does our blood provide oxygen and nutrients for all our body parts, it also picks up carbon dioxide and other waste matter to be disposed. This is handled by our heart—our main pumping station.

Although the heart is only about the size of a small fist, it is the most important organ in our body. It pumps life-giving blood into small tubes that we call "arteries." The arteries divide into even smaller tubes, called "capillaries." The oxygen and food nutrients cross the capillary wall and feed the body cells. While there, they pick up carbon dioxide and waste, which are then carried back through the capillary wall into the blood.

Our capillaries join together to form veins. During the alternating oxygen/waste process, waste material is picked up and transported by the blood through the veins. When the blood reaches the heart, the process starts over again. The heart is divided in half, with two chambers on each side. One is called an "atrium," which receives blood and the other a "ventricle," which pumps blood out. The blood carrying waste from the veins enters the heart through the right atrium, and is pumped through the right ventricle and into the "pulmonary" arteries to the lungs. Once there, the blood collects oxygen and releases its carbon dioxide. Then it is pumped back through the pulmonary veins to the left atrium, down to the left ventricle then out through the main artery, called the "aorta." From there, it feeds the body again, and the circle is now complete. All this work in just THIRTY seconds! Do you suppose that if we took the time to breathe more deeply, in a clean and fresh environment, and put the burden on the diaphragm, instead of the heart, that maybe our hearts wouldn't have to work so hard? Hmmm…

The next area of the body that we need to take a look at is our digestive system. It's one of the largest systems, and it spans about thirty feet from mouth to anus. In order for the food we eat to be converted into nourishment for our cells, it must be broken down. The whole process starts in the mouth. After the food is chewed, it mixes with our saliva. Good digestion starts with chewing long enough to allow the saliva to do its job.

Just before we swallow, a small flap called the "epiglottis" shuts our windpipe off, so that food doesn't enter the lung and we don't choke. The food then passes down the esophagus into the stomach. Once there, the food churns with our stomach acids and is broken down into liquid form. The liquid then passes into the small intestine. At the same time, our liver manufactures a green digestive juice, called bile. The bile is then sent to the gall bladder to break down fats. Meanwhile, the pancreas is producing digestive juices, plus insulin to lower our blood sugar and to turn off our hunger signal.

All the digestive juices then mix with the broken-down food in the small intestine. Once there, the mixtures slip through the intestine wall into the blood. The remaining water and undigested food then passes into the large intestine. There the water is absorbed into the blood and is passed on to the urinary system, while the solid waste is stored and finally pushed out through the anus.

Although we appear to be solid, our bodies are actually about seventy percent water, which must be balanced everyday. We usually take in approximately two-and-a-half quarts of water daily through our food and drink. We lose about a quart just through breathing and perspiring, and we lose the other one-and-a-half quarts through urination. The job of the urinary system is to filter the waste from the blood. It does that by forcing the blood through the kidneys up to five hundred times every day! The kidneys are about the size of a fist, and shaped like a kidney bean.

Just like the heart, the renal arteries push toxic blood into the kidneys and the renal veins remove the clean blood. During the filtering process, a watery fluid is formed called "urine," which is passed through two small tubes called "ureters," to the bladder where it is stored. When the bladder is full, it contracts and pushes the urine out of the body through a tube called the "urethra."

Which brings us to the reproductive system. Although it is different in men and women, basically they are similar and interconnected. In females between the ages of 11 to 52, every month her ovaries produce the hormone "estrogen," which releases a ripe egg into a fallopian tube where the egg can then be fertilized. If the egg is fertilized, it grows and continues down the tube into the "uterus," or womb. Once there, the egg nestles into the uterine wall, where it gestates for about nine months, and a baby is born. If the egg is not fertilized, then the lining of the uterus and the egg are released through the vagina. This process is called the menstrual cycle.

While the female reproductive system is hidden inside her body, the male reproductive system is on the outside. Between his thighs hangs a pair of egg-shaped testes in a sac called the scrotum. From about the age of thirteen or so, the testes produce testosterone and sperm. The sperm, which look like mini tadpoles, are stored in a long tube called the "epididymis," and are carried in the sperm duct to the prostate gland. The prostate then supplies a liquid in which the sperm can travel down the urethra and through the penis to fertilize an egg.

When we examine our nervous system, we find that it is the body's electrochemical communication network. It's the highway that allows the body parts to talk to one another. The nerves run throughout the body, carrying messages through the spinal cord and to the brain, which is the major organ of the entire system and the body's control center. In an average adult, the brain weighs about three pounds and it contains about ten thousand, million nerve cells. It is responsible for thought language, emotion, and memory. The brain is also divided into three parts: the cerebrum, the cerebellum and the brainstem. The cerebrum is the largest part of the brain and is divided into two sections called "hemispheres". The right hemisphere is usually associated with creativity, and the left hemisphere is associated with numbers and logic a la Mr. Spock. The cerebellum is responsible for muscle movement and posture, while the brainstem controls all the vital, involuntary actions, such as breathing and heartbeat. Our nervous system is so fast, that it sends messages across our body at about one hundred-eighty-five miles an hour, a feat that would certainly warm the cockles of any race car driver.

Lastly, we have our senses of sight and sound. The eye is the organ of sight. It rests within the bony sockets of the skull, called orbits, and it is protected from the outside by eyelids, eyebrows, and a thin film of tears. It is connected directly to the brain by the optic nerve. Each eye is moved by six muscles, which are attached around the eyeball. It works like a camera. The light enters the pupil and is focused by the cornea and lens into an upside down picture on the back wall, called the retina. The retina can sense light and color, and can convert the picture into electrical impulses, which it sends across the optic nerve to the brain. The brain then turns the picture right side up.

The ear is the main organ of our sense of sound. The sound waves collect in the ear and pass across the auditory canal to the eardrum, which makes it vibrate. The vibrations then travel across three tiny bones: the hammer, the anvil and the stirrup, which turn the waves into electrical signals. The electrical signals are then shot across the auditory nerve and picked up by the brain for interpretation.

The human body is a miraculous machine and it would take years to fully understand it. Basically, these pictures are only here to help you familiarize yourself with the shape and location of your problem areas. Since you are about to take your own fantastic voyage into your own body, I just thought that it might be a good idea to know where you're going and what to look for. You don't have to be that accurate. A simple picture in your mind representing a bone, an organ, or a body part is more than sufficient. Remember, it is intent that really counts here.

**Today's Date** _____

# FUNSHEET #3

## Visualization #3 – Talking with your Body

**Pain/Negativity Levels**

0 - Completely calm/relaxed/pain free

1 - Feeling tense/tired/slightly uncomfortable

2 - Some agitation/nervousness/discomfort

3 - In stress/pain apparent

4 - Agitated/throbbing pain

5 - Highly agitated/unbearable pain

**Locations of Discomfort/Stress   Pain/Negativity Level**

|  | *Before* | *After* |
|---|---|---|
| 1) _____ | 0 - 1 - 2 - 3 - 4 - 5 | 0 - 1 - 2 - 3 - 4 - 5 |

**What did you first see?** _____

**What is it feeling?** _____

**What color was the energy face?** _____

**What's wrong?** _____

**What does it want?** _____

**Information received:** _____

_____

_____

_____

As you can clearly see in Funsheet #3: *Talking With Your Body*, I have used the same pain / negativity scale for you. This time, I suggest that you choose no more than two body parts to work on. As a matter of fact, on your first try, I suggest that you do only one. Write the name of the body part that is challenging you the most next to the number one under Locations of Discomfort & Stress. Decide how much it is bothering you and choose a number from zero to five, according to the pain / negativity-level scale, then circle that number under Before.

Please take a minute to read the questions. These are the same questions that I will be referring to in your visualization. "What did you first see?" The first thing you want to take note of during your visualization is the outside of the organ or body part that you're looking at. Check out its texture. Is it shiny and smooth, or dry and pitted?

What about its color? Is it dark or light? Does it have spots of color on it? Is it ashy looking, or brown, blue, pink, orange, yellow, or red? What is it feeling? Is that body part exuding a recognizable emotion like sad or angry, bitter, cautious, or is it happy and loving?

Ask the body part to tell you what's wrong? Is it a life circumstance, or something simple, like not paying attention to the body part's needs? What does it want? If you listen very carefully here, your body part will tell you what to do to correct the situation.

The "information received" lines are for comments or suggestions made by your body part. Fill them in after your visualization.

Are you ready? Record the following visualization or pop in CD #1 and go to Track #3 -*Talking With Your Body*, and have a relaxing, good time. Now, remember not to get too comfortable. You need to stay alert and awake. Catch you later!

## Visualization #3 – *Talking with Your Body*

Get into a very comfortable position. Place the tips of your thumb and index fingers of each hand together to form a circle and make the okay sign. Keeping your fingers in the okay position, turn your hands palms up. Now rest them either on top of or along side your legs. Now close your eyes. Begin to drift with the music as it gently flows over you.

Imagine a large blackboard in front of you. Inhale deeply. Hold the breath *(for the count of 7).* Exhale slowly. See the numbers 3, 3, 3. Inhale. Hold the breath *(for the count of 7).* Exhale. See the numbers 2, 2, 2. Inhale. Hold the breath *(for the count of 7).* Exhale. See the numbers 1, 1, 1.

You are standing in the hallway of a very posh hotel on the 10th floor in front of the elevator. Press the elevator call button. The doors open and you step inside. Select the lowest button. It is four floors below the 1st floor. The doors close. Now watch the lights above the doors as you begin to descend.

10 going down, 9 further down, 8 quiet, 7 relaxed, 6 tranquil, 5 silent, 4 serene, 3 calm, 2 harmonious, 1 love, PP peaceful place, lower level A, automatic bodily function, lower level B, body rhythm, lower level C, central body command.

The doors open into an underground system much like the subway. As you step outside the elevator doors a most unusual vehicle is parked there for you. It is bright and shiny and shaped like your favorite car but it floats on air. It has no wheels. It is fully automated and runs on voice command so you don't have to steer it.

Now step inside your vehicle, sit down and buckle your seat belt. Tell your vehicle to take you to the point of discomfort or illness. *(pause)*

Your vehicle begins to float down a bright green tunnel. It picks up speed. It bypasses the tissues of your body and goes further down to the cellular level. It quickly comes to a stop in front of the body part that is giving you difficulty.

Look through your windshield and examine that body part thoroughly *(pause)*. Can you see anything wrong with it? *(pause)* What is it feeling? *(pause)*

Your vehicle shrinks down a bit and takes you directly into the body part. You can see the cells moving around. It goes a little deeper now into the atoms, protons, neutrons, electrons and into the space between. In that space between the atoms there is a swirling color forming the shape of a face. Take note of that color. *(pause)*

Flip open your communication switch on the control panel of your vehicle. Tell your body part that you are sorry for causing it so much trouble and ask what's wrong. *(pause)* Find out what it wants. *(pause)* Tell it you will be happy to do that. *(pause)*

If it's been hurting you, ask it if it can stop. *(pause)* Tell it to please do so immediately. *(pause)*

Now ask any other questions that you wish. *(pause 60 seconds)* Thank it for taking the time to communicate with you and promise to love it. *(pause)*

You may now start your journey home or tell your vehicle to go to another body part and start asking the same questions there. *(long pause - two minutes)*

Thank your cells for talking to you. *(pause)*

It is now time to tell your vehicle to take you home. Your vehicle turns around and goes back up through the cells. Up through the tissues and into the green tunnel. It continues its journey upward through the tunnel and comes to a full stop right outside the elevator door. *(pause)* Open the vehicle door. *(pause)* Step outside. *(pause)* Close the door behind you and walk to the elevator. *(pause)*

Now push the elevator call button *(pause)*. Watch the doors open. Step inside and press the number 5. At each number you will become more and more alert. One, beginning to come up now, two, becoming more alert, three halfway home, four, almost there, five, open your eyes, fully awake and feeling great.

## Funsheet Reminder

I hope you remembered to completely fill out your last Funsheet. If you haven't, please take a moment to do so right now. The reason I stress that you do this immediately after your visualization is because in a few moments, you may not remember what occurred during the visualization. In a few years, you'll never remember what insights you were given or how changes occurred during this healing process. You may very well be in the middle of a true medical miracle right now, and will never be able to show your doctors how you got here because you didn't document it. It's important that you keep accurate records so you can track your progress.

When I found myself wrestling with cancer, I kept a log of every supplement I took, every herb, everything I ate, and every unusual occurrence and piece of information I received. By the way, I neatly handed this log over to my doctor when it was over and didn't make a copy. I worked very hard and had a diary to prove it. There is also another reason for you to journal these visualizations, you will need the information for your letter "E": your Evaluation process. When you've finished your Funsheet, go back to your house of well being chart and your goal sheet, and put the information you just received where it belongs. You may now have a vital piece to your illness puzzle. Then put it on your "to do" list.

# Chapter 6

## Connecting With Your Higher Wisdom

## More of Letter "H"

The following visualization is the core to everything I've been sharing with you: there is a way to connect with that part of you that has all the answers. It goes to the biblical promise that, "Before you call, I will answer." Now, think about that for a minute. What if Creator / God / Goddess were standing right in front of you? What mysterious secret would you want to know the answer to? What problem would need solving? What miracle would you ask for?

Well, here's your big chance. You are about to tap into that Higher Wisdom that is part of all of us. Actually, you have already been doing this from different angles since we started. Your Higher Wisdom is in every cell and every energy particle in your entire body. First we used it to relax our body and to balance our chakras. Then we used it to stop pain. Then we traveled to the actual body parts, and now we are going straight to the heart of the matter.

By that, I mean the part of you that lives in a small pocket behind your heart, commonly referred to as your soul. It is the child of your larger spirit, which encompasses all of you. To put it another way, your soul is your memory bank, your subconscious mind. It remembers every thing you have ever said, done, or experienced, in any dimension across time. It also has access to the Akashic records, which is commonly called the "Book of Life," or "God's Book of Remembrance. " You might say it is the universal library, which contains the unlimited knowledge of Creator. I've come to believe that our soul already knows what our conscious mind cannot even fathom.

Since I realize that you could have a million questions on as many different subjects, I decided to use this visualization as an exercise to help you discover which diet or foods should be included or avoided in your new health program. Once you have gotten that information, feel free to use this visualization at any time to answer any question on any topic

## Basic Nutrition

It's pretty much common knowledge that the more fresh fruits and vegetables we eat, the healthier we are, and the less likely we succumb to serious disease. Then why is it so hard for most of us to eat right? Well, the answer might lie in our family upbringing, which guided our personal preferences. For instance, if you grew up in the South, you may have eaten everything fried and with gravy. If you grew up in the Midwest or the North, like I did, you probably were introduced to hearty foods, like red meats, soups, and stews to keep warm. In the West and Southwest, you probably ate more dishes with cheese and spices. In any case, we are a product not only of our family, but of our geographic location, as well.

As a matter of fact, there is a whole eating plan called Macrobiotics, which advocates eating food grown in the region in which we live. Since our bodies are part of the energy fields around us, the local plants best support them. Eating foods that are home grown is simply healthier for us because nature put them there to help meet our climatic needs.

To better understand what we are to eat, maybe we should start with what the body actually needs, and that is vitamins, minerals, and amino acids. Since each of these plays its own unique role to our overall good health, we're going to have to take them one at a time from the following list.

# Vitamin Chart

| Name | Type | Description |
|---|---|---|
| A | Fat Soluble | Needed for digestion of protein, rebuilding organ tissues, teeth and bones. Prevents night blindness. As an antioxidant, it helps fight cancer. |
| Bs | Water soluble | Calms nervous system. Fights stress, fatigue and depression. Metabolizes fats, carbs proteins. Nourishes brain cells and builds red blood cells. |
| C | Water soluble | Stimulates immune system to ward off infections. Lowers cholesterol. Heals wounds, burns and bleeding gums. A vitamin C flush cleans intestines and sparkle the entire body. |
| D | Fat soluble | Needed for calcium absorption, strong bones, teeth and proper sleep. Helps reduce stress and boosts the immune system. |
| K | Fat soluble | Needed for blood clotting and converting glucose into glycogen, which helps prevent osteoporosis. |

We start with Vitamin A, which is also known as Beta Carotene and belongs to the fat-soluble vitamin category. That means that it can be stored and need not be taken every day. Your body needs Vitamin A for the secretion of gastric juices that aid in the digestion of protein. This vitamin also rebuilds organ tissues, teeth and bones. Along with Vitamin C, it helps fight infections and viruses and prevents night blindness. It is also an antioxidant, which helps fight cancer. Vitamin A is commonly found in things that are orange and yellow, like apricots, carrots, cantaloupe, fish-liver oils, animal livers, and green and yellow vegetables. Vitamin A is usually paired with Vitamin D.

The B-Vitamins work together and are water-soluble, that means that any excess B Vitamin in the body is automatically excreted and not stored by the body; therefore, it must be replaced daily. We need the B-Vitamin group for a healthy nervous system, as well as for fighting stress, fatigue, and depression. They are also necessary to nourish our brain cells and to metabolize fats, carbohydrates, and proteins. Without our B-Vitamins, our hair won't shine, our nails break, our skin ages, our gastrointestinal, or GI tract becomes weak, and we become anemic. We also need Vitamin Bs to keep Candida in check and for the synthesis of cortisone, insulin and sex hormones.

Anyway, according to Dr. Balch, in his book *Prescription for Nutritional Healing*, our best sources of B-Vitamins are brown rice, dried beans, egg yolks, fish, liver, fresh fruits and vegetables, dairy products, nuts, soy products, and whole grains. However, Vitamin B-12, which is necessary in the prevention of anemia, is not found in vegetables. It can only be found in meats, dairy, and seafood.

Vitamin C is also a water-soluble vitamin, and it must be replaced every day. We need Vitamin C to ward off infection, to lower our cholesterol, to stimulate our immune system, and to protect us against stress. This vitamin also helps us to heal wounds, burns, and bleeding gums. It can also have a laxative effect when taken in high dosage, which is sometimes called a Vitamin-C flush. Some holistic practitioners recommend a flush when fighting unknown viruses, or to clean out our intestines. Vitamin C can be found in citrus fruits, like oranges and grapefruits, lemons, pineapples and strawberries. It can also be found in green vegetables as well as tomatoes, onions, papayas, rose hips, and currants.

When we combine Vitamin C with Vitamin E, the effect is greater than taking them separately. In combination, they are powerful free-radical fighters. Ester C, in particular, was found by Dr. Jonathan Wright to increase our white cell count four times more than regular Vitamin C. This is great news for patients suffering with AIDS, cancer, and other chronic illnesses.

I've always wondered why Vitamin D is called the "sunshine" vitamin. Now I know why. Dr. Balch says that the ultraviolet rays of the sun can be converted to Vitamin D within our body. In supplement form, however, it requires conversion by the liver and kidneys before it becomes fully active. Personally, I'd rather take a healthy walk in the sunshine once in a while rather than take a pill. In any case, we need Vitamin D for proper sleep, for strong bones and teeth, and for good calcium absorption, to prevent osteoporosis. It also helps us to reduce stress, and it enhances our immune system. We can get our Vitamin D from fish liver oils, fatty saltwater fish, like salmon, eggs, and dairy products fortified with Vitamin D. It can also be found in alfalfa, butter, cod liver oil, egg yolks, halibut, liver, milk, and oatmeal.

There has been much written about Vitamin E over the last few years, especially about helping to heal scar tissue. It too is a fat-soluble vitamin and can be stored. We all need Vitamin E for lubrication of our joints and bones, but it is also known for its antioxidant properties that help prevent cancer and cardiovascular disease. Vitamin E also improves circulation, repairs tissue, and is sometimes used in treating cysts and PMS. It promotes healing, clotting, reduces blood pressure, and assists with leg cramps. But most importantly for us beautiful females, it helps retard aging. In order for us to keep good levels of Vitamin E in our body, we must be supported by the proper level of zinc.

Lastly, we come to Vitamin K. What makes vitamin K so important is that without it, our blood won't clot and we become bleeders. It also converts glucose into glycogen, which is stored in the liver and plays an important role in keeping our bones healthy and in preventing osteoporosis.

# MINERAL CHART

| Name | Type | Description |
|---|---|---|
| Sodium<br>Potassium<br>Calcium<br>Magnesium<br>Phosphorus | Macro (bulk) | This group of minerals is needed in large quantities by the body for balancing the systems, rejuvenating the organs and accelerating cell growth.  . On the cellular level, an imbalance in minerals is one of the basic causes of diseases. |
| Iron<br>Zinc<br>Copper<br>Chromium<br>Manganese<br>Selenium<br>Germanium<br>Molybdenun<br>Silica<br>Sulfur<br>Vanadium<br>Iodine<br>Boron | Micro (trace) | This group of minerals is responsible for the proper function of the chemical and electrical processes that are occurring at every moment within your body |

There are two of minerals groups: macro (bulk) and micro (trace). Bulk minerals are needed in large quantities by the body and include: sodium, potassium, calcium, magnesium, and phosphorus.   Trace minerals include: iron, zinc, copper, chromium, manganese, selenium, germanium, molybdenum, silica, sulfur, vanadium, iodine, and boron.   They can be purchased in powder, tablet, and capsule or in chelated, liquid, colloidal, ionized forms, which are easier to absorb.

While the human body can manufacture vitamins from the foods it ingests it cannot create minerals. Minerals must be obtained from outside sources and are a requirement for optimum bodily function.

Now that we understand the role that vitamins play in our body, let's take a look at minerals. Without minerals we do not get the proper absorption of our B-Vitamins. In addition to being necessary for the balancing of our body fluids and our hormones, we need minerals for energy, and to quiet our nerves. Without minerals, we have poor blood, weak muscles, including the heart, and dry hair. Minerals are also necessary for a strong immune system, and to regulate the pH of our blood, either acid or alkaline. Normal blood is slightly alkaline. That means it is above seven on the pH scale, and it usually reads somewhere between 7. 3 and 7. 45.

Some physicians, like Dr. Joel Wallach, who is not only a naturopath but who started out in the regular medical community as a veterinarian, believe that mineral deficiency is the cause of most chronic illnesses today, like diabetes and arthritis. In his many years of practice, in case after case study, when minerals were introduced to sick patients, the improvement was remarkable. Dr. Wallach and his colleague, Dr. Ma Lan, have written a great book called *Let's Play Doctor*, which can help you immensely in taking control of your own health. If you want to hear more about the importance of minerals, as well as have a great laugh, try to get Dr. Wallach's tape, *Dead Doctors Don't Lie*. I can assure you, you're in for a great treat.

## 10 Essential Amino Acids

These are the building blocks of protein, which are needed to repair and re-build all bodily functions. They are - arginine, histidine, isoleucine, leucine, lysine, methionine, phenylamine, threonine, tryptophan and valine.

The last category of nutrition that we are going to cover is amino acids. They are the "building blocks" that make up the protein in our food. There are twenty-nine amino acids that make up all living things. About eighty percent of those are produced by the liver but there are ten called essential amino acids that are not made by our bodies and must be obtained through the diet. They are: arginine, histidine, isoleucine, leucine, lysine, methionine, phenylamine, threonine, tryptophan and valine. Whew! Tryptophan—that's the easy one. It's the one in turkey that helps us fall asleep after Thanksgiving Dinner.

Without getting too technical, amino acids are essential to the rebuilding of all cells in the body. Without amino acids, our central nervous system shuts down because it doesn't receive information for our neurotransmitters. Simply put—our brains turn to mush. But most importantly, without amino acids, all the vitamins and minerals we eat will not be absorbed and assimilated.

At the present time, there is a whole new field of medicine that is being born. It is called "metabolic" or "functional" medicine. The doctors are finding out that by taking a simple stool analysis and amino acid test, they can find out what your body is missing. They are now also able to link amino acid deficiency with certain behavior disorders. My mild-mannered husband had become extremely irritable, flying off the handle at the slightest annoyance. His amino acid test showed that he was low in tryptophan, which is needed to promote serotonin in the brain. His doctor ordered two amino acid IV drips. As soon as he finished the drips, changed his diet, and started taking the necessary supplements, boom—he was back to his normal, calm self.

Which can bring us to a very simple conclusion. We must eat a balanced diet: two to three servings of protein, two to three servings of fruits, four to six servings vegetables, two servings of fat, and one to three servings of complex carbohydrates, like brown rice, sweet potatoes, and whole grain products. Now remember, potato chips are not considered a vegetable. Stay away from empty junk foods, and just walk a few blocks a couple of times a week. If we eat different fruits, veggies, and proteins every day, then the variety will take care of all our nutritional needs. If we don't balance our diet, we may have to supplement to get what we're missing from our food. It's not that complicated. There are dozens of books and hosts of dietitians and nutritionists who can help. Check your local directory or log on the internet, or just go to the local library or health food store and start reading. You may find out that your particular illness can be greatly improved or healed just by adding a particular food to your diet.

Following is a suggestion from my angel guides as to what constitutes healthy proportions for daily maintenance of health and weight.

## Angel Food Tray

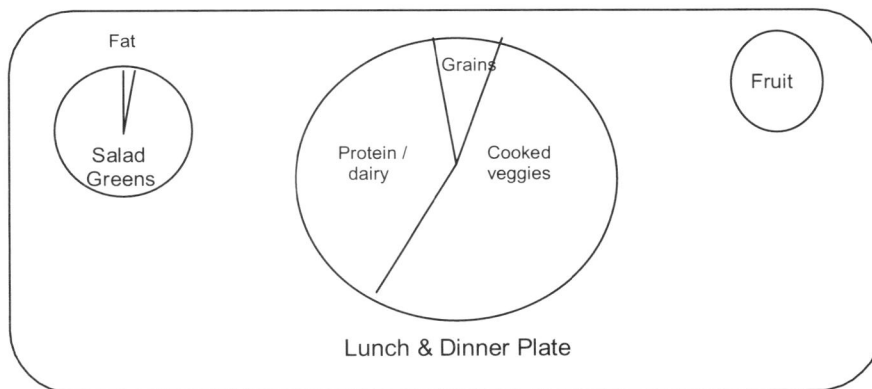

Fat

Grains

Fruit

Salad
Greens

Protein /
dairy

Cooked
veggies

Lunch & Dinner Plate

As far as diets go, there are many different philosophies. One of those is simple Food Combining. You may find that food combination charts are all that you need. Or better still, check out one of Suzanne Sommers' books. My favorite is *Eat, Cheat and Melt the Fat Away.* She has become an expert on the subject and her recipes are great.

If that doesn't suit you, or if you want to get more detailed, there are several Exchange List Diets. Dieticians commonly use them in hospitals and they usually follow the food pyramid philosophy.

Then there is Macrobiotics, which is the oriental art of balancing the energies in the body, called the "yin and yang." Interestingly, the name Macrobiotics came from Hypocrites and is Greek. "Macro" means large or great and "bios" means life.

Another diet philosophy that is practiced in India is called Ayurveda, which means the "science of life." It is built on three metabolic principles called "doshas." The doshas govern the flow of intelligence throughout the body. If you wish to find out more about Ayurvedic medicine and diets, check out Dr. Deepak Chopra's books and his tape *Perfect Weight*.

With the understanding that cooking depletes vital nutrients out of our food, almost all the philosophies and nutritionists stress the importance of keeping our fruits and veggies as close to raw as possible. When I was trying to win my own battle with cancer, my healing angel suggested a vegetarian diet that was ninety percent raw. In the past few years, when I have asked for the best diet for a particular illness, I wasn't surprised that my answer was usually either ninety percent raw, seventy-five percent raw, or fifty percent raw. I have outlined those diets here to help familiarize you with the concept. They are by no means a solution to your individual needs. However, they could be a starting point for you. You might wish to include them in your visualization, and / or review them with your health care provider to see if any one of them might be of some benefit. You may want to check out Ann Wigmore. She has written several books on raw food that provide excellent information and insight.

Here is a simplified list of a few diets you may want to review before you do your next visualization. You may be guided to choose one of these to jump-start your healing process. They differ from the above Angel Food Tray in that these are geared to cleansing the body to allow it to heal faster. They have more fiber from vegetables and fruits and most of the protein suggested is from nuts and seeds rather than animal. In this manner, the body rids itself of unwanted accumulated debris that may be interfering with recovery.

## Diets for Healing

## Vegetarian Diets
*(Contains nothing having eyes)*

### Diet A – 90% Raw

| Breakfast | Fresh fruit |
|---|---|
| **Lunch** | Large salad sprinkled with raw, unsalted nuts/seeds for protein |
| **Dinner** | Small salad with nuts/seeds plus some steamed vegetables |

### Diet B – 75% Raw

| Breakfast | Fresh fruit |
|---|---|
| **Lunch** | Large salad sprinkled with raw, unsalted nuts/seeds for protein |
| **Dinner** | Small salad with nuts/seeds, steamed vegetables, ¾ cup brown rice |

### Diet C – 50% RAW

| Breakfast | Fresh fruit plus cooked whole grain cereal (oatmeal, barley, bulgur, grits, buckwheat, etc.) with a splash of rice, soy or almond milk. |
|---|---|
| **Lunch** | Large salad sprinkled with raw, unsalted nuts/seeds for plus 1 cup fresh vegetable soup with miso/tofu or legumes. |
| **Dinner** | Small salad with nuts/seeds plus some steamed vegetables, ½ cup cooked legumes, ¾ cup brown rice or any whole grain or baked sweet potato (not white). |

## Animal Protein Diets

*(No more than four oz. of meat/fish/poultry per day range fed and purchased at a health food store)*

### Diet D - 30% Raw with MEAT

| Breakfast | Fresh Fruit plus cooked whole grain cereal (oatmeal, barley, bulgur, grits, buckwheat, etc.) with a splash of rice, soy or almond milk. |
|---|---|
| Lunch | Large salad sprinkled with raw, unsalted nuts/seeds for plus 1 cup fresh vegetable soup with miso/tofu or legumes or two ounces of lean meat/fish/poultry. |
| Dinner | Small salad with nuts/seeds plus some steamed vegetables, ½ cup cooked legumes, or two ounces of lean meat/fish/poultry, ¾ cup brown rice or any whole grain or baked sweet potato (not white). |

### Diet E - Combination Vegetarian and Animal Protein Diet

You may eat two vegetarian meals and save your four oz. of meat for either lunch or dinner.

### For All Diets

No coffee, tea, sugar, white flour products, breads, yeast, heavy spices, commercial salad dressings, butter, dairy products, eggs, or white potatoes. Use lemon, brown vinegar, olive oil for dressings. Mashed avocado with tomato (guacamole) is OK. Nothing is to be fried. Dried fruits may be used as snacks in small quantities if they are raw and unsulfured.

Remember to choose a diet that is not only the best for your condition, but that suits your lifestyle. Don't be afraid to make changes if necessary.

Sometimes one diet will work for a couple of weeks and then we have to change to another.   As our body changes, so does our chemistry and its nutritional requirements.

The following Funsheet will be used for your next visualization.   This time we're going to concentrate on our solar plexus and brow area.  Take a minute to check their sensory or intuitive levels, and mark the corresponding numbers under the "Before" column.  After you've completed that, I suggest that you choose these first three questions to clarify your diet.  Do this by the process of elimination.  You could start out by asking, "What type of diet should I be on now - meat, vegetarian or combo? "  When you get that answer, then you could ask: "Which philosophy is best—Food Combining, Exchange List, Macrobiotic, Ayurvedic, or Percentage of Raw Foods? "  After that answer, you may want to go to, "How long do I need to be on that program—one week, two weeks, three weeks, or longer?"  In that way, you know that you need to check back in a little while to update.  You may want to ask questions like, "Is there a particular food that I need to be eating now, and for how long? "  Or, "Is there anything that is presently in my diet that I need to avoid completely, and for how long? "  In that way, you'll know that the change is only temporary.

Another subject which could be very beneficial to you are questions regarding cleansing.  By that I mean, is it necessary that you clean out and detoxify your body at this time?  There are many types of cleanses which could be done like short juice fasts, an herbal tonic, or a "colonic. "  Although there could be great benefits gained from cleansing, it should be done under medical supervision.  I highly recommend that if your Higher Wisdom suggests that you do a cleanse, that you contact your physician or health care provider and check with them before making any attempt.  Not only could you experience serious side effects and not know how to handle them, over-cleansing can be downright dangerous.

I think you get the idea about your questions, so start your Funsheet now, record the following script or pop in your visualization #4.   You'll find it on CD #1, Track 4 - *Connecting With Your Higher Wisdom*.   When you're finished, write down your answers and comments.

## Visualization #4 – *Connecting with Your Higher Wisdom*

Get into a very comfortable position place the tips of your thumb and index fingers of each hand together to form a circle and make the OK sign. Keeping your fingers in the OK position, turn your hands palms up.  Now rest them either on top or along side your legs.  Now close your eyes.  Begin to drift with the music as it gently flows over you.

Imagine a large blackboard in front of you.   Inhale deeply.   Hold the breath *(for the count of 7)*.   Exhale slowly.   See the numbers 3, 3, 3.   Inhale. Hold the breath *(for the count of 7)*. Exhale.   See the numbers 2, 2, 2.   Inhale. Hold the breath *(for the count of 7)*.   Exhale.   See the numbers 1, 1, 1

You are standing in the hallway of a very posh hotel on the 10th floor in front of the elevator.  Press the elevator call button.  The doors open and you step inside.  Select the button that is one below the first floor.  It is marked PP. The doors begin to close.  Now watch the lights as you begin to descend.  10, going down, 9, further down, 8, quiet, 7, relaxed, 6, tranquil, 5, silent, 4, serene, 3, calm, 2, harmonious, 1, love, PP, peaceful place.

The doors open to the most beautiful peaceful place you can possibly imagine.  The trees are lush and green.  The sky is blue.  The sun is shining. There are birds singing and the air is fresh and sweet.  As you look forward, right in front of you is a yellow brick path.  It is called the road to clarity.  To the left of the path is a body of water.  It is your favorite body of water.  There is a light mist in the air from the water and it gently caresses your face.

To the right of the path is a beautifully landscaped garden.  It is full of your favorite flowers.  Go over and smell the flowers. *(pause)*  They are bright, vibrant and pungent. *(pause)*  It is time to leave the flowers and walk up the yellow brick path.

At about 15 paces the road splits into three forks. Each fork has a directional sign. One points to the left. One points straight ahead and one points to the right. Take the road straight ahead, the one that is marked "Window."

Walk about 20 paces and you will see two trees. They are your favorite trees. Slung between the trees is a hammock. Go and lie down on it. Gently sway back and forth. Back and forth. So quiet. So peaceful. So restful.

Visualize a brilliant golden light shining down from the trees. *(pause)* As it comes closer to your face, it spins in a counter-clockwise direction like a small tornado at the top of your head. Now it spreads out into a pyramid shape beaming its golden light onto the center of your forehead. *(pause)* It feels warm and tingly. You are filled with a sense of wonder and feel pleasantly lightheaded. *(pause)*

Turn your attention for a moment to the edge of the hammock close to your right hand. Hanging from the edge is a small silver cord. Gently give it one tug. *(pause)* Continue to relax and enjoy this marvelous peaceful place.

Turn your attention back towards the top of the trees. As if by magic, the most magnificent picture window slowly descends. It is the window of knowledge. This window is surrounded by a hand-carved, gilded frame. The window comes down and stops right in front of your face. You can easily peer into it. Through the window you can see a beautiful angelic being. This is your Higher Wisdom. Take a minute to greet and experience the compassion and beauty of your love essence. *(pause)* Now ask your first question and wait for your answer. *(pause 60 seconds)* Ask your second question and listen for your answer. *(pause 60 seconds)* Now ask your third question and wait for your answer. *(pause 60 seconds)*

Thank your Higher Wisdom for all its help and say your good-byes. *(pause)* Allow your right hand to reach for the silver chord and this time give it two gentle tugs. *(pause)* Your window now slowly goes back up into the trees. *(pause)*

The golden light over your head begins to swirl again, this time in a clockwise direction. It lifts and spins up back through the trees into the clouds *(pause)*. Now swing you feet from the hammock back to the ground. *(pause)* Stand up and start walking back up the yellow brick path toward the elevator. Pay close attention, as you are walking, to the trees, the water, the gardens. This is your beautiful peaceful place and you can come back here anytime you wish. *(pause)*

You are now back in front of the elevator door. Turn around one more time and etch this place in your mind, its sights, it sounds, its smells, its feelings, its warmth and its love. *(pause)*

Now turn around and press the elevator button once more. The doors open. Step inside and press the number five. The doors close. At each number you will become more and more alert. One, beginning to come up now, two, becoming more alert, three, halfway home, four, almost there, five, open your eyes, fully awake and feeling great.

**Today's Date** _____

# Funsheet #4

## Visualization #4 – Connecting with your Higher Wisdom

**Intuitive Levels**   0 - None
1 - Feel mild sensation/presence but cannot identify
2 - Feel a medium sensation and some identification
3 - Feel a strong sensation and can identify easily

## Locations of Intuitive Centers          Intuitive Level

|  | *Before* | *After* |
|---|---|---|
| 1) Solar Plexus _____ | 0 - 1 - 2 - 3 | 0 - 1 - 2 - 3 |
| 2) Brow _____ | 0 - 1 - 2 - 3 | 0 - 1 - 2 - 3 |

## Personal Questions

1) _____
2) _____
3) _____

Answer to #1)

_____
_____

Answer to # 2)

_____
_____

Answer to # 3)

_____
_____

## Comments/other recollections:

_____
_____

If you still have unanswered questions, please do the visualization again and again, if necessary, until you get them resolved. Sometimes answers bring on even more questions. It's just a matter of elimination and perseverance. Remember, this is a skill-developing program. Eventually, you'll be able to take any piece of music that makes you comfortable, go to your alpha level with the techniques you've already learned, and ask as many questions as you like on any topic that is relevant to your situation and your Highest Good. By that I mean, anything that benefits the growth of your soul. Unfortunately, asking for lottery tickets and numbers usually doesn't belong in that category.

The last subject I'd like to talk about is herbal medicine. For thousands of years our eastern cultures and our own Native American culture used nature's pharmacy to heal their people. It has only been in the last couple of decades that we have moved away from the fields and into the laboratory. The good news is that with all the advances in western medicine technology, we now have the ability to pinpoint a diagnosis with great accuracy and to operate on almost any body part. The bad news is that, oftentimes, we're too quick to cut, and pass up the opportunity to save an organ because we're ignorant in matters of natural therapies.

That task falls to us, not just to become educated in herbal substitutes for traditional, over-the-counter remedies, but to help our physicians become educated as well.

I believe that Dr. Andrew Weil has the right idea. On one of the talk shows he said that Western (allopathic) and Eastern (homeopathic) medicines need to be integrated, so the patient can have the best of both worlds. He was the first to coin the phrase "Integrative Medicine", which is alive and continues to attract a growing number of physicians today. Furthermore, he also said that natural remedies should be encouraged and used about eighty percent of the time and pharmaceuticals and surgery the other twenty percent. If we can keep that type of balance in medicine, we'd probably all live longer, healthier, and more fulfilling lives.

As I've said before: read, read, then read some more. Anyone who has healed themselves from anything will probably tell you that they researched their illness from many angles, then took what they thought was best for themselves. There are many good books on herbal medicine to choose from in your library and your local bookstore. My favorite is *Natural Healing with Herbs* by Humbart Santillo because it is easy for me to understand, but you need to find the ones that "speak" to you.

Again, I caution you not to take anything without consulting a physician that is well versed in herbal medicine. Just like prescriptions, herbs can react with other herbs and other pharmaceuticals. It's best to get someone who is well versed in both modalities. If there is no one in your town, try looking on the internet. You can also write to the American Medical Association, either in Chicago or Washington, D. C., and the American Association of Naturopathic Physicians in Seattle, Washington. If you find a doctor that is on both lists, you may have yourself a rare find!

Of course, the most important part of your health regime should be prevention. Eating right, exercising, getting enough sleep and taking at least three time outs each day for peace and quiet is paramount to any health program. I urge you to make them a part of yours.

# Chapter 7

## Body/Mind Connection
## More of Letter "H"

Although there has been a lot of talk about the Body / Mind Connection, it suddenly occurred to me that experiencing it could better serve us here. So let's take a minute to try a simple exercise. I'd like you to stand in front of a mirror with your eyes closed. Point your chin slightly upward toward the ceiling, and replay in your mind the funniest incident or joke you ever heard. Got it? Pause for a few seconds then open your eyes and look quickly in the mirror. Are you smiling? Are you standing tall? Did you laugh? How did that make you feel? Did it uplift your spirit? Did your tummy move up and down? Was it a real belly laugh? I want you to hone in on all of those feelings.

Now, let's try it again. Only this time I want you to replay the saddest moment of your life. Once you have the image and the feeling, open your eyes and glance at the mirror. Is your face different? How about your posture? Did it bring tears to your eyes? Was the feeling heavy? How did you experience that idea?

Congratulations! You have just experienced the body / mind connection first-hand. I want you to get this, because a very important principle is about to unfold here. You see, not only does the body follow the mind, but the emotional body follows the mind as well. We talked about that before, when I mentioned Dr. Burns' book, *Feeling Good*. First comes the thought, then comes the feeling, then comes the change in the body. But what none of the doctors or psychologists has been able to explain is—why? For that, we have to take a peek at who we truly are.

In Neal Donald Walsch's *Conversations with God*, he gives new meaning to the Trinity with these aspects. I've expanded a little on Neal's thoughts and created a visual tool to help you understand more fully. Read this chart one line at a time from each box. Start at the uppermost level of the center box (Spirit) then the uppermost entry in the lower left box (Mind) then the uppermost level in the right lower box (Body).

## Three Aspects of Life

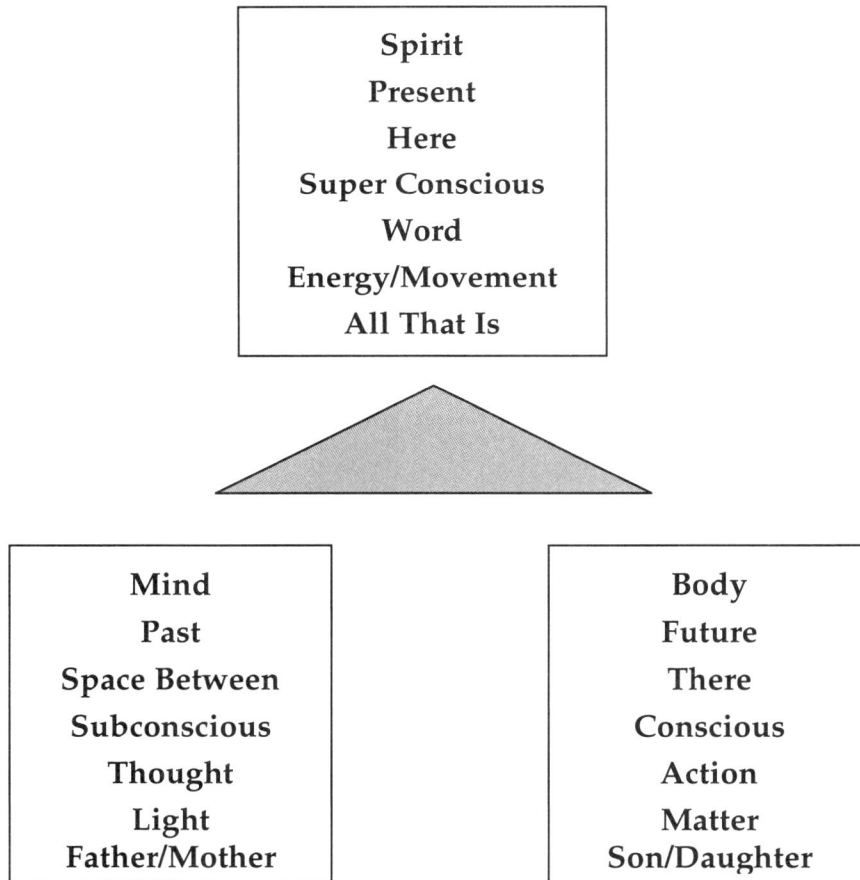

**Spirit**
**Present**
**Here**
**Super Conscious**
**Word**
**Energy/Movement**
**All That Is**

| **Mind** | **Body** |
|---|---|
| Past | Future |
| Space Between | There |
| Subconscious | Conscious |
| Thought | Action |
| Light | Matter |
| Father/Mother | Son/Daughter |

Here you can see the correlation, under the individual headings. Normally we read them as: body-mind-, past-present-future, here-there-space between, conscious-sub conscious-super conscious, thought-word-action, energy/movement-light-matter, All That Is-Father/Mother-Son/Daughter.

As you can see, every part of our three-dimensional world is made up of three aspects. If you start with the words at the top of each box, you can see that man is a "tri-une" being—having a mind, a body, and a spirit. On the next level, that which we call time is also divided into three categories: past, present and future. Distance can be measured as here, there, and the space between. Awareness is measured in conscious thought, subconscious thought, and super consciousness thought. The three aspects of creation are thought, word and action.

Let's talk about that for a minute. It appears that everything that has ever come into our world started with a single thought that was either spoken or written down as a word or as a drawing. The combination of thought and word then moved it into three-dimensional matter.

Here we can see what many of us have been taught about our Creator. Namely, that He or She also has three aspects, commonly referred to by Christians as Father, Son, and Holy Spirit. In Hinduism, which is the oldest religion on the planet, those same three aspects were called Brahma, Shiva and Vishnu.

Interestingly, in Hebraic tradition, although there was no mention of three aspects, there was mention of the masculine aspect Adon, as in the word "Adonai"—meaning Lord or Ruler—and the feminine aspect, which was called the "Shekinah," and represented earth and beauty. In fact, there are presently many rabbinical scholars who believe that the Old Testament was written by two authors—one feminine and one masculine—which may account for the different ways in which God is portrayed in the Old Testament. On the one hand, God is loving and kind and, on the other hand, as vengeful and angry. If you're interested, you can read *The Book of Jay*.

In any case, if we look up or down the list of our chart, the parent aspect—as in father, mother or both—also can be called "thought," as in "in the beginning," which puts it in conscious mind, here in the present. The Holy Spirit, commonly depicted as a white dove, is considered by some to be the feminine aspect of God—the Goddess—and can also be called "the word." It holds all memories of the past in the subconscious, and is the space between here and there. It is also the internal spirit of man. The Son aspect can be the embodiment of one person, as in Jesus of Nazareth, or it can simply be God in body form, as in all mankind, or both. Your interpretation depends on what your heart and awareness says right now. So choose the one that is most comfortable to you. If you look up the line, the Son aspect can also be the result of action, the higher or super consciousness that only knows love, the end of the destination as in "there," and the shining future as well as the body of man.

There you have it—God omnipresent and omnifarious. That means God in all things. Think of it this way - water is always water, but it comes in many forms: vapor, snow, hail, ice or rain. Each molecule is the same, but they bind together differently and change form as the temperature changes.

What I truly want for you to get from this exercise is this most important understanding. Do you remember the biblical phrase: "and the word was made flesh"? What if we took that literally? Since word can either be spoken or written, when we take a thought, then add a word, then add an action, we create a baby. By that I mean, we create a living breathing creation in our world. Now, I'm not talking about a person, although one would have to have a thought about making love, convey that to his or her partner, and then go into action for that to occur. What I am specifically talking about is bringing into being a new drama or a new object, like the invention of the telephone, the automobile, or the computer. Every man-made thing that we touch in our world started with a thought, then a word or a drawing, then some kind of effort to get it off the ground.

In the same way, so did all our experiences. First we got a thought, such as, "I hate my job. I think I want a new career. " Then we spoke our idea to someone who pointed us toward a direction, then we went into action by getting some training, or we wrote a resume and went for an interview, and hopefully got the new job. If we examine it very carefully, everything that has ever happened in our lives followed the same formula—thought, plus word, plus action.

Now here is the tricky part. Since we are made in the image and likeness of our Creator, and were promised by our Team Captain that, "Before you call, I will answer"—is it possible that God has been reading our thoughts, then answering us either in experience or through others, in accordance with what we have been saying in our own everyday speaking? If that were true, then when you speak, God speaks, and when I speak, God speaks, and when God speaks—So It Is. If I continue to say "I'm sick" or "I'm tired," then maybe in my own speaking, God answers, and I continue to inadvertently create the experience of feeling more sick and tired. Maybe the way to avoid this is to keep my words in check. Better still, what if I wanted to turn it around? What if I were to say, "I'm getting better and better, stronger and stronger. " As Jose Silva suggests in his Silva Mind Development program, could that help turn around my illness? From my own experience, I believe it can.

I'm not referring to keeping a positive attitude. An example of positive attitude is a situation where your cat accidentally poops on the rug one second before the doorbell rings announcing the arrival of your dinner guests. You quickly run and put a flowerpot over the mess and keep a positive attitude that no one will notice. The problem is that the smell is still there. Positive thinking will not get to the root of the problem.

What I am referring to when I say, "It is so important that I watch my words," is that the energies of thought and word are the first two levels of creation. If I literally don't want my words to come back to haunt me, the first thing I must learn to do is to monitor what I am saying about the illness I'm focusing on healing. If I name it, like "my arthritis" or "my diabetes," then I have claimed it. It's mine forever. If I don't want that illness to continue in my world, it would then be best for me not to give it the power of my words, or any power at all, for that matter.

I know this is difficult. It took me almost eight years to figure it out after I heard it from my first healing teacher, Karmelia. She was trying to get me to see the body / mind connection in helping me to heal manic depression. She said, "From now on, stop saying you're manic. " I listened to her but, truthfully, I had no clue as to why she was saying that to me. It wasn't until I read Neal Donald Walsch's *Conversations With God: Book 3* that I finally got it. (By the way, I highly recommend you read his books when you get a chance.) It was, as Oprah would say, a "GE moment. " The light bulb went on, and I had this most crucial and final piece to this program. When we put the three aspects of creation together—thought / word / action—a result can form in our physical body. This is commonly referred to as the mind / body connection. The energy of thought first creates an emotion, then the emotion affects our hormone flow, and the result is a change in our body.

Getting back to understanding the thought / word / action principle of creation, I have a simple homework assignment for you. For the next three days, pay close attention to the speaking of everyone you come into contact with in your world: your family, your friends, your coworkers. Just listen to how they talk about their life. Are they always complaining and seem to have more trouble then they know what to do with? Are they doubtful and are always forced into making decisions? Or are they happy and speaking as though everything is okay?

Once you get the knack of listening, I'm sure that not only will you see the connection of what they are saying as to what is happening in their world, but you will also be able to pick out their illnesses. If they are unbending or critical in the speaking, then look for stiffness in their body, like back, neck, or joint problems. If they are always worrying, look for heart, circulatory, or stomach problems. If they are always angry or disgusted, look for something red and swollen inside or outside, like ulcers, carpal tunnel, acne or arthritis. If they can't find the sweetness in life and want to control everything their way, look for diabetes.

You get the idea, but please, please don't say anything to them. It is not for us to judge or condemn others for making the same mistakes that maybe we ourselves have made. They will come to you when you get better and ask you how you did it. That is the time to share your new truths. You can even suggest that they get this program. Hey, a little advertising doesn't hurt.

I share this very important information with you because for me it was the missing link to all my sickness. When I stopped speaking as though I were sick, I stopped feeling sick. When I stopped feeling sick, my thoughts moved away to more creative places. I just reversed the process!

Maybe Jesus said it best. In three simple sentences, he told us that we had this great power to change our lives and where it came from. He said, "Why are you so amazed? Even greater things than I have done, so shall you do" - Greater than changing water into wine, raising the dead, or walking on water? What can be greater than that, and why is it that he expected us to do this? I think that answer lies in his third sentence, when he said, "The Father and I are one, and you are my brethren. " If we are all his brothers and sisters, and we all came from the same source, it's not such a stretch to believe that we are all one with the Father. If we are all one with the Father, then, of course, we have the power to do great things. But how do we do them? Maybe the same way the Father did—by putting thought, word and action together to move "God energy" into the physical world.

What would be a great thing in your world right now? Wouldn't getting completely healed from your illness or life situation be a great thing for you?  Sort of a new person would be born out of that experience.  I've given you a lot to think about.  I suggest that you pray or visualize on what I have just shared with you.  These are my personal truths.  I invite you to find yours.

What I want you to get out of all of this is that there is not just a body / mind connection, but a body / emotion / mind connection.  If we don't address the emotional body's connection to the onset of disease, then we cannot completely heal.  Why?  Well, my healing angels were kind enough to set me straight.  They say, **"The body follows the mind, provided the emotional body concedes. "**  That's why you haven't been able to heal even though you've been taking medicine and supplements and doing everything right.

That's very powerful.  That means that the root of all sickness lies in the emotional body.   You probably haven't addressed the emotional body.  Some doctors know this.  They tell us that most illnesses are caused by stress.  Unfortunately, there is no prescription that can eliminate stress.  We must do it ourselves.  Where does stress come from?  Well, it comes from what we say about the circumstances of our life and from our thoughts.  Our thoughts come from what we believe.  What we believe comes from our past.  And what came from our past is probably no longer serving us, except to make us sick.

If we continually re-create our past and bring it into our present, we literally have no future.  That's like doing the same thing, over and over and over again, the exact same way, and expecting to get a different result.  It just won't happen!  Someone went so far as to call that behavior the definition of insanity.

So what are we to conclude from this?  If the body will follow a more positive mind, provided the emotional body concedes, then it's up to us to absolve and clear the emotional body at the same time that we are absolving and clearing the physical body, or at least as quickly as possible.

How can we do this?  Well, we can go into therapy for the next twenty years like I did or we can get a fresh perspective, one that will help us shift and release those trapped feelings.  That's why I'm creating a library under the logo *Angels to the Rescue*.  My challenge in writing this program was to help you through the emotional healing process without being physically present.  It would be very easy if you were sitting in my office and we went through your angers and your fears and your guilt's.  But in good conscience, I could not send you to face any of those emotions alone, so I called upon the "E-lo-him" to help out.  The Elohim are the Archangels whose ranks have ascended in consciousness from third dimensional thinking to unconditional love either when visiting our planet or in other realms.  They are also known to some as the Masters of the White Brotherhood not because of the color of their skin but because of the white robes they wear.  Since membership includes both males and females from every philosophy, every culture and race since the beginning of time and some are unknown to us, we agreed to now refer to them as the Masters of the Family of Light.  In either case, they agreed to help out and here we are.

Before we can absolve and cleanse the emotional body, we need to dissect it.  In Chinese medicine, the major organs of the body are directly connected with particular emotions: the heart with joy and sorrow, the lungs with worry and grief, the liver and gallbladder with anger, the spleen and pancreas with sympathy, and the kidneys with fear.

In western medicine, these factors have been left to the psychologists.  So what makes up the emotional body?  I like Dr. Elisabeth Kubler-Ross's teachings best.  They were re-iterated by Neal Donald Walsch in his *Conversations With God: Book 3*, and deserve another look right here.  Dr. Kubler-Ross said that everybody has five natural emotions.  They are: love, fear, grief, anger and envy.  When these emotions are expressed naturally, there are few repercussions in our life, but when we suppress them, they wreak havoc in our lives, and in our bodies as well.

Let's take these emotions one at a time.  Love is a normal and natural emotion.  When children play, they like to touch and be close to everybody.  They express love without embarrassment, limitation, or inhibition.  When a parent cuddles or plays with a child, he/she receives love.  But when children are taught not to get close or not to break the rules, or not to express their love or mommy will be upset, they begin to think that expressing love is not okay.  They experience the withholding of love from a parent and at the same time force themselves to repress what is natural for them.  They interpret love withheld as meaning they are not worthy of love.   Thus, they grow up having a difficult time expressing and receiving love as adults either repressing and having a cold exterior or becoming overly promiscuous.  Such repressed love turns into possessiveness, a very unhealthy and unnatural emotional state.  Possessiveness can land in the solar plexus and give you ulcers and other digestive disorders.

Fear is also a natural emotion.  We are all born with the fear of loud noises and a fear of falling.  This was the gift of self-preservation.  However, all other fears in our lives are either instilled in us by our parents, teachers, society leaders, religious leaders, media are simply created in our imagination.   If children feel that it's not okay to express or experience their normal fear, they squelch it and have difficulty expressing it in adulthood.  Repressed fear turns to panic, and panic creates arrhythmia in the heart.  Any wonder why heart disease is so prevalent in America?  High stress is caused by fear of losing family, friends, home, job and possessions.

Grief is also a natural emotion.  It allows us to express sadness at a time of loss.  In fact, it doesn't have to be the loss of a loved one; it can be loss of a job, or a pet, or even the experience of losing our place in society.  Retirees often experience this when they leave their position in the working world and are no longer in powerful company positions.  Suddenly some are reduced to being old folk playing on the golf course.   When children are encouraged to cry and let their grief out, they get over it quickly.  But when they are taught that it's not okay to cry and they have to take it like a man or be strong, they later have a hard time expressing it when they are adults. Grief that is stuffed down and repressed becomes depression. The hospitals are filled with people who suffer from unresolved grief. Not only does it affect our mental state, but it also can be the cause of some cancers. It also impacts the pelvic chakra region, and can be responsible for elimination and reproductive disorders.

Anger, when recognized as a response to a person or circumstance that did not live up to our expectation as way for us to learn to better communicate or say "No" or to set boundaries, is a very natural emotion. If children were taught to set boundaries and not expect people to always be perfect and do exactly what they say they are going to do, they would not have unreasonable expectations of others or become abusive or hurtful adults. Anger that is bottled up and not cleared through communication easily turns to rage. Rage turns into diseases that are inflamed, red and swollen, like arthritis, carpal tunnel, and severe acne.

Now envy is a little tricky. We've all experienced the feeling of wanting something that someone else has, but envy is also the emotion that drives us to try harder and to reach farther. You might say that it is at the core of friendly competition. Children who are allowed to express envy and experience it are able to move through it quickly as adults. But adults who harbor envy turn it into the green monster known as jealousy. There have probably been more wars over jealousy than any other emotion. Jealousy can attack your throat chakra and tighten your voice, your lungs, and your chest.

Basically, all our emotions were given to us as gifts to empower us. They are yardsticks for us to measure the difference between this experience and that experience. This experience makes me feel happy. That experience makes me feel sad. By pointing out the differences, our emotions are supposed to guide us into choosing the more loving and comfortable of the two feelings. That is what self-love, or taking care of ourselves is all about!

Unfortunately, if we were never taught that emotions are simply yardsticks for experiencing the circumstance of the moment, we could find ourselves labeling some emotions "good" and others "bad." In actuality they are neither good nor bad. They are simply feelings given to us that assist in interpreting our present state of being. In not wanting to experience or express the "bad" emotions and allowing them to pass quickly, we stopped loving ourselves. On the day we stopped loving ourselves, our illness was born. Creator God/Goddess/All That Is —that which we are part of and who only knows Love—cannot be sick, cannot be broke and cannot be dead. We literally pull ourselves away from our own natural instinct of self-love and self-expression by stuffing down the emotion of the moment and not moving through it. Unfortunately it has no place to go.

We **are** love in our true essence. Negative emotions are not to be harbored inside us forever. They belong outside the body as part of universal energy, where they can be transmuted back into love. When we continually hold onto negative energies derived from collective emotions, we stay sick.

# Chapter 8

## Absolving/Clearing the Emotional Body
## Letter "A"

Now that we know what makes us sick, how do we heal the emotional body? Simple - we absolve it to clear out all the negative energy that is keeping our illness going, and then we re-balance it back to the state of Love. As I said before, the best way to do that is to get a different perspective on the situation. In that way, the negative energy starts draining out.

How do we do that? We open up our heart to feel, our third eye to see, and our crown chakra to connect and communicate. Here are the eight steps that I use to incorporate those three aspects. .

### Eight Steps to Healing the Emotional Body

Step 1: Get calm and centered. Take some deep breaths. Inhale to the count of eight. Hold for the count of eight then exhale for the count of eight. You can also still your chattering mind by simply telling it to stop. Saying something like, "Mind be still and know that I am love. " Then follow with a short prayer, like, "I am one with the light; I am one with my angels. "

Step 2: Call forth all the incidents that created your emotional energy blocks, one at a time. In the beginning I do not recommend doing more than one. Remember that these are emotional incidents that need to be cleared. You may cry or experience a wide range of emotions. We're all different. Whatever happens will be unique to you. When you are more experienced, you can ask your angels simply to give you a list of all the incidents or people you need to look at. You know, sort of a "To Do" list. Then choose one at a time when you are ready, and clear them out individually.

Step 3: Try to find the good that came about. Loretta LaRouche one of our great spiritual humorists calls this finding the "bless in the mess". You can do that by looking at the incident through the eyes of the other person or people involved. One technique that I've used is to say, "Show me the heart of so and so at the time of the incident. " I remember the first time I did this. I was shocked to find out that the other person involved never really meant to hurt me. The hurt that I experienced came from the conclusions that I had drawn, and what I had said about the person and the incident! All of the unhappiness came from my personal perspective. I highly recommend that you rent the documentary movie *What the Bleep Do We Know,* which explains the new phenomena of quantum physics as it relates to our individual perspectives of life. It's not just fascinating but the cartoon characters and special effects make it a lot of fun to view.

Step 4: Ask your angels for clarification. That will get easier and easier as you practice. You'll be amazed at how much love you will feel when you finally get connected and your angels can communicate with you. Since they are able to give us a more loving look at the incident, and help us to see it from the other's point of view, they can also help us get through the next step very quickly.

Step 5: Forgiveness. Forgive him or her or them, and then forgive yourself. It's very important that you include yourself in the forgiveness process: forgive yourself for holding onto these negative feelings for so long, and for your part in the drama. Once we have forgiven all those involved in our incidents and have forgiven ourselves, the negative energy is released, and we go into what I call the "healing mode. "

Step 6: Release the negative energy back into the Universe. You can do this by seeing it as smoke rising, then turning into violet particles of light that dissipate into the sky. Or better still, take a deep breath, then blow it out.

Do that three times and you'll feel a whole lot better.

Step 7: Balance your chakras. Now, that will create a new and more balanced energy flow in your body. And finally…

Step 8: Say a prayer of gratitude. Not only is it important that you acknowledge your angels, your Creator, or whomever you are working with for their assistance, but it also sets the stage for the reversal of disease. My favorite prayer is, "Thank you, God/Goddess for my radiant health. "

## Dissolving Guilt

When I talked to my healing angels about this program, they told me that although there are five natural emotions, there are only three that have to be dealt with specifically—guilt, anger and fear. Since guilt is the easiest one to tackle, I chose it to be first.

When I think of guilt, I immediately think about all those chocolate donuts I ate when no one was watching. They, along with my favorite pasta dishes, helped bump me up to "fluffy but fabulous. "

Alas, my angels have another view of guilt. They say guilt is part of a formula: **Contradiction** plus **Justification** equals **Guilt**. The contradiction part means going against your own personal truth or belief system. So when you contradict or go against your own truths or beliefs, and then try and justify doing so, you end up feeling guilty.

Let's see how the formula works with my chocolate donuts. My personal belief/truth about food would be something like: "Healthy people avoid sweets and high calorie foods and they don't cheat on their diet. " When I ate the donuts anyway, I justified doing that by saying, "But I need something sweet. I'll cut back tomorrow. " That's when I felt guilty. Sound familiar?

Now, let's try the formula once more, only this time, let's add another person into the mix. Here's the scenario: You tell your mother that you're working on Sunday and you can't come to dinner, when you are actually going out with friends. If you hold a belief like, "good children don't lie to their mother," or, "I don't lie, period" and then you justify the lie by saying, "Well, I had to do that, because if I had told her the truth, I would have hurt her feelings," you are going to experience some modicum of guilt.

Now those are minor guilts, you know, cheating on a diet or telling a white lie. But what if someone you loved died, maybe in an accident where you tried to help but were too late? If, in that case, you held the belief that, "Good people don't let their loved ones die," or, "I don't stand by while someone is dying," then you justify your behavior during the incident by saying, "but I wasn't strong enough," or, "I couldn't get there in time," you are probably carrying a very heavy load right now.

What if someone you know died during a serious illness? Are you saying things to yourself like, "I could have done this, or I should have done that? " Or, "if only…" The psychiatrists say that the words "could a, would a, should a" will keep us locked in guilt for a lifetime if we continue to use them. Is that where you want to stay?

I'd like to put this type of guilt to rest here and now, once and for all. Guilt that is born out of the so-called untimely demise of someone in our world comes from us not knowing the most important Universal truth. Before I tell you what that truth is, I'd like to walk you through it first. Now I know that I'm going out on a very long limb here, so please let this scenario sink in before you make any judgment about the messenger. You don't have to agree with me. All I'm asking you to do is to consider the possibilities.

Here's the scenario. A junkie goes into a liquor store to hold it up. He pulls out a gun and says to the shopkeeper, "Empty the drawer. This is a hold up. " While the shopkeeper is taking the money out of the cash register, a policeman just happens to walk in the store. The officer immediately knows what is going on draws his weapon, and shouts, "Stop! Drop your weapon. This is the police!" The junkie gets frightened and shoots the shopkeeper. The police officer immediately shoots the junkie. Both the shopkeeper and the junkie are now lying dead on the floor. The question is: "Who's a murderer? "

Society would say that the junkie is a murderer because he took the life of another while committing a crime, but the cop was only doing his job. However, the junkie and the shopkeeper are both dead. From this example, it would appear that the word "murderer" is merely a label we choose to put onto somebody, depending on our judgment of the act and not on the act itself. In our civilization we have many occupations besides being a police officer that could involve the taking of a life. There are soldiers in battle, CIA or FBI agents protecting our country, and doctors caught between saving one life or another.

Now, let's go back to the holdup scenario and take it one step further. The two bodies are lying on the floor. The souls separate, come out, and go wherever they go. Now tell me—who died? That's right—no one!

Now here comes the tough part. My master teachers say, "There is no person on the planet that is ever responsible for the death of another. " Why? There are four reasons.

#1: As we just figured out, there is no such thing as death. There is only a transition from pure positive energy, physical, into pure positive energy, non-physical. We, our energy and consciousness, live forever. Granted, in the example, the junkie and the shopkeeper are not here on the earth anymore, but they are alive and well and living somewhere.

#2: You and I do not have the power to obliterate the forever existence of another soul. Only God can do that, and a loving God never would.

#3: By the co-creative power of God that is part of who we are, each one of us calls our own shots. We control our own destiny, not another's, no matter what the circumstances, the condition of the body, or the age, be that one minute or one hundred years. To cite that point: have you ever heard of an infant that had been badly beaten or burned, and left to die in a garbage can, that was found and miraculously survived? The soul of the infant did not want to leave, and chose to have the earthly experience, possibly of disfigurement, rather than leave, even though an adult made the attempt to send it off.

#4: All that we call murders are simply staged dramas, accomplished by agreement between souls for a higher purpose. Those souls logged the request and final agreement in the Akashic Records. As I said before, the Akashic records are the files known as God's Book of Remembrance.

Think of it as a big book or computer database in the hereafter. The Akashic Records are located on the 33rd Dimension also known as the 33rd Plane of Consciousness. Before we come here, we visit the Akashic records to choose our parents, design our body, outline or detail our life, and write our name. That's right—we choose our own name and then inspire our parents to give it to us. We can also request extremely difficult life or death challenges, which require a partner, a volunteer to be carried out. Why? For the experience itself. You see, we cannot come to love, compassion, and understanding of another until we've walked a mile in his shoes. To that end, I guess in one lifetime or another, we've all been murderers, rapists or thieves. It certainly doesn't boost our ego any to admit that, but how else can we find out what it's like to be on the other end? You tell me.

I didn't like it either when I first heard it. You see, my whole world was based on Conditional Love. And Conditional Love is based on judgment. I only love you "if" - If you think like me, if you are good, if you do as I say, and so on. In other words, I don't love you unless you measure up to what I believe that you should be.

It took me a long time to make peace with that most difficult Universal truth I alluded to earlier. Here it is: **"There are no accidents, no victims, and no villains. "** Everything that has ever happened, is happening now, or will ever happen, is in Divine Right Order.

In order to accept that concept, I had to move to the possibility that there is such a thing as Unconditional Love: a love that is given freely without any judgment whatsoever.

Now I know that is a tough one to swallow, but please remember I'm only the messenger here. I too have had loved ones assaulted and leave this earth through tragedy. My own son died in a jet-ski accident, went to the light, and mercifully came back. I personally have been robbed, beaten, molested, date raped and almost killed a few times in this lifetime, and I tell you, it's no fun. But within the depth of my being, I know that all these experiences made me strong and brought me here to these pages, today, to assist you. I also know that on a higher level, my soul called forth those experiences without notifying my conscious mind. I would have chickened out. I, therefore, have to accept that my spirit was a willing participant in all those dramas. I played good guy to somebody else's bad guy. But as sure as my name is Annemarie, I also know that there is someone out there who would say that in his or her eyes, I played bad guy to their good guy in some encounter that we may have had.

To illustrate the good guy / bad guy syndrome, or the differences between shadow and light, let's take a look at a high-profile murder. Have you ever thought that maybe the O. J. trial was necessary to help us evolve spiritually? How? Did that case not help us put race issues on the table, so that all of us could have an opportunity to recognize and clear our own prejudices? Did it not help battered women to start standing up for themselves? Didn't shelters spring up all over the United States, and weren't the abuse laws toughened? What I'm trying to help you see is that some good comes out of even the worst tragedies.

Even the survivors of Hurricane Katrina have raised the consciousness of the nation. Did we do right by them? Will they be caught up in a political battle or will they fight to rebuild their beloved cities and re-structure the political system that let them down? We don't know where that is going to lead us at all. The really sad part about all of these disasters is that it always takes a huge incident before we make things right in our world.

Unfortunately, it appears that in the course of human history, there has always been a tragedy before a triumph. Maybe it's the way we have chosen to learn.

I truly believe that the souls of those who made their transition in all those types of incidents, as well as those who committed the so-called crimes, did what they did to advance their own soul growth and, at the same time, volunteered to teach us something. This is a grand sacrifice and should not be simply dismissed as tragedy or the lunacy of a few disturbed citizens.

By the same token, those who have left the planet in natural or man-made disasters, such as war, have also left their mark behind for us to re-group and make changes. Those who made their transition via the Titanic incident changed the maritime laws. Those who suffered and left in concentration camps showed us how love could flourish even in this most noxious of environments and dramatically illustrated the folly of prejudice. All of these souls are to be honored. They helped us see value and beauty of all races and religions.

And those who made their transition through earthquake, flood, hurricane and volcano helped us to clean up the earth, and forced us to change our building codes while protecting our environment. They also gave us opportunities to explore our own courage under disaster, and to start new lives by learning to let go of all our earthly possessions.

Maybe we should just say "thank you" to those who have blessed our lives with their suffering and their sacrifice—a sacrifice that helped us to open our eyes to change what needed to be changed.

If we come to accept that there are no accidents, no victims and no villains, and everything is in Divine Right Order, we come to understand we have been sitting in judgment of all the people and incidents of our life by labeling them good or bad, right or wrong. It is these judgments that make up our belief system. When we realize that it is not the people or the incident itself, but our judgments that have created our way of being, we then have a

110

strong base to forgive each other and ourselves for acting human. We may also come to realize that what we call our earthly life is merely an illusion played on a grand stage with other actors to help us evolve spiritually. After all, through unconditional love all roads lead home, whether through light or through shadow.

Without accidents, victims or villains, there's no reason to feel guilty, unless we keep holding onto a personal truth that chocolate donuts are evil. I choose to believe that our Creator made us in His/Her image to prosper, grow and evolve into the light of pure love by whatever means we desire. I also believe that Creator is merely an observer and chooses for us what we choose for ourselves. That is what is called Unconditional Love and it comes with the gift of free will. Ultimately, it's up to us to choose who we want to be and what we want to experience to challenge that choice. But in order to choose a way of being, there must be choices. As the song says "I can be happy or I can be sad. I can be humble or I can be bad. It all depends on me. Oops! I'm showing my age.

Please understand that I am not advocating the murder of innocents, the bombing of buildings, or the theft or destruction of property by anyone at anytime. This is not the Wild West. We don't take the law into our own hands and we don't need to steal or kill to eat. We have all kinds of social programs to handle that in case someone truly can't pay for food. We have evolved past stealing and killing types of behaviors. We're into a new way of being.

According to my healing angels, man's inhumanity to man shall no longer be tolerated here on the earth. You might say that the shadow element is making its last stand before leaving here forever. This is what I believe the second coming or new age is all about, relinquishing judgment to make room for the Christ.

Christos is a Greek word that means " useful good; anointed, master of love. " Now is the time for the coming forth of the Christ that lies within all of us.  Each of us is becoming our own master of love.  To be in alignment with that path, I am asking you to find the good in all things, even the horrors of our world, and learn to forgive those who appear to be in shadow.

When we judge others, it is because we see in them a part of ourselves we don't like.  We measure them by a yardstick that even we can't reach.  When we label another "murderer, rapist, thief, stupid, selfish, careless, or mean," we actually unleash and send the negativity or shadow element that lies within us out into our own world.  We then feed it with more judgment, and it comes back to bite us "you know where. "  These same labels swirl around in our head and we wind up using them as a weapon to judge ourselves.  It's time for us to evolve and to stop that kind of thinking and speaking.  It's time for us to walk our Love talk.  And, more importantly, it is time for us to choose whom we want to be - Enlightened or Un-enlightened?  The word enlightened means "to be in light of; to have knowledge. "

Choosing enlightenment is accepting ourselves - our shadow and our light without judgment and striving to be our highest ideal.  When we can love all that we are, we can then extend that love to another without judgment.    The new millennium is the time to abandon the Age of Victimization and enter the Golden Age of Love.   Be the light of your Creator.   Shine for everyone that crosses your path.   A smile can save a life.  A touch can lift despair.   A word can heal a body and a look can spark great change.

I'd also like to address one other issue.  Sometimes when people first grasp the concept that we are all part of Creator, and that Creator doesn't make mistakes, which is why there are no accidents, no victims and no villains, they immediately go on another guilt trip.  "Oh my gosh, I can't believe that I brought all this misery on myself.  I did it.  It's my fault. "  Please don't go there.  It's not my intention to lay that on you. Understanding that you can be in control of your own world is an opportunity to empower you.  You are now sitting in the driver's seat and can, therefore, make better

112

conscious choices. That is what empowerment is all about: an opportunity to change your world for the better by staying in your peace, and calling forth your spirit to guide you in all things. This should be empowering, not dis-empowering. When you start blaming yourself or someone else for the circumstances of life, you actually dis-empower yourself. You give up your God power and slide into shadow. The result is you diminish who you truly are.

To be clear on all that I have said on guilt, all we have to do is go back to our formula: Contradiction + Justification = Guilt. That means when we act in a way that is contrary to our own personal beliefs, then justify doing that, we will feel guilty. To stop feeling guilty, you either have to stop justifying your behavior or change your belief system. It's that simple. If you choose to change your belief system to unconditional love and extend that love to yourself and your own actions, you will never again have to justify them and, therefore, will never feel guilty.

Enough said! It's time to let go of whatever guilt you may have collected. It no longer serves who you are becoming. You may not even consciously know that you have any guilt, but I assure you, odds are that there is some hiding down in your lower chakras. You won't know until you lift up the rock and look under it, so either record the following visualization or pop in CD #2 – Track #1 *Dissolving Guilt* and then fill in the following Funsheet.

## Visualization #5 – *Dissolving Guilt*

Get into a very comfortable position and place the tips of your thumb and index fingers of each hand together to form a circle and make the okay sign. Keeping your fingers in the okay position, turn your hands palm sides up. Now rest them either on top of or along side your legs. Now close your eyes. Begin to drift with the music as it gently flows over you.

Imagine a large blackboard in front of you. Now inhale deeply. Hold the breath (*for the count of 7*). Exhale slowly. See the numbers 3, 3, 3. Inhale. Hold the breath (*for the count of 7*). Exhale. See the numbers 2, 2, 2. Inhale. Hold the breath (*for the count of 7*). Exhale. See the numbers 1, 1, 1

You are standing in the hallway of a very posh hotel on the 10th floor in front of the elevator. Press the call button. The elevator doors now open. Step inside. This time press the button that is one below the 1st floor. It is marked PP. The elevator doors close. Now watch the lights above the door as you begin to descend. 10, going down, 9, further down, 8, quiet, 7, relaxed, 6, tranquil, 5, silent, 4, serene, 3, calm, 2, harmonious, 1, love, PP, peaceful place.

The doors open up onto the most breathtaking peaceful place you can possibly imagine. The sun is bright. The sky is clear blue. There are several giant puffy white clouds floating overhead. The air smells so sweet and the dew so fresh. There are birds in the trees. You can hear them singing merrily.

In front of you is a yellow brick path. It is called the Road to Clarity. To the left of the path is a body of water. It is your favorite body of water and there is a cool mist in the air and it brushes your face.

To the right of the yellow brick path is a garden full of your favorite flowers. Bend down and smell the flowers. They are colorful and smell so wonderful. Ask the bushes if you may pick a flower. Watch for them to giggle. It's your sign that it's okay. Now pick two of the most beautiful blooms. Thank the bush for its gift. Now start walking up the yellow brick path.

At about 15 paces you will come to three directional signs. One points to the left, one straight ahead and one to the right. Take the path in the center, the one marked "POOL," and start walking straight ahead. Continue walking. Observe the birds and the small animals scurrying about. Admire the beautiful trees and foliage on each side of the path.

At about 20 paces you will come to a white chain link fence. Walk to the gate. *(pause)* Waiting at the gate are two beautiful angels, one male and one female, each holding a shepherd's staff. They open the gate for you. Greet your angels and hand each one a flower. *(pause)* Introduce yourself and ask him or her to speak their name or to write it on the sign-in book on top of the white pedestal inside the gate. *(pause)*

One of your angels hands you a shopping bag with a special gift inside and instructs you to open it later. Thank them for the gift, then hang the shopping bag on the gate knob for you to pick up later.

Your angels begin to give you a guided tour of this breathtaking pool. Although it is man made, it was designed to be part of nature and is nestled close to the base of a small mountain. The pool is edged with natural rock and landscaped with trees, flowers, and tropical plants, each having been especially selected and planted here just for you.

On the shallow end there is a natural waterfall from the mountain. Your angels motion you to follow them to the right side of the pool. Once there, they climb up three stone steps, then turn right and sit on a bench that overlooks a natural lotus pond. The water is crystal clear with beautiful flowers floating towards its edge. You can easily see your reflection in the water. Take a seat in the space they have left for you in the middle of the bench. You are now sitting between your angels.

This is the Pool of Recollection. If you ask a question and then toss an object into the pool, the answer will appear when the ripples stop. The answer could be in the form of a picture, a voice or familiar sound, a written word or simply a feeling of knowingness.

Now turn to your angels and ask them to show you the incident that resulted in the guilt you have been harboring in your body. *(pause)* Take a deep breath and as you exhale, begin to focus your attention on the center of the pool. One of your angels touches the tip of their staff into the water to create the ripple. It is now beginning to clear. Stay focused on the center. *(pause)* You are receiving the information very clearly now. *(pause)*

Now turn to your angels and ask them, "Did any goodness or blessings come from this?" *(pause)* "How can I grow from this experience?" *(pause)* "Am I not responsible? *(pause)*

Turn to your angels and ask them if there is anything else you have to see. If they say yes, tell them you will come back next time. *(pause)* Thank your angels for their assistance. *(pause)*

Your angels begin to rise and motion for you to follow them to the shallow end of the pool. *(pause)* Step into the water and walk under the waterfall. Watch as your angel raises his or her staff and touches the falling water. It immediately changes to a cooling mint green color. As the water begins to wash over your body from head to toe you begin to experience a cleansing, cooling, freeing sensation.

Now repeat after me in your mind. "Beloved Creator, with Your healing waters, I hereby wash away and release all the guilt, all the negativity and all the resulting disease I have created. I now change my reality. I thank you for my newfound radiant health. So be it and so it is. AMEN

Stay in the waterfall until you feel completely cleansed. *(pause)* Step out from under the waterfall into the sunlight. Look up through the clouds and see the face of your Creator smiling back at you. *(pause)*

It is time to leave the pool area and say goodbye to your healing angels. Follow them back to the gate. *(pause)* Say your farewells. *(pause)* You may wish to give them a hug. *(pause)*

Don't forget the shopping bag with your gift. Pick it up and wave goodbye as you start walking back up the yellow brick path towards the elevator door. At the left side of the door is a small bench. Go and sit on it. *(pause)* Now reach into your shopping bag and open your present. Examine it carefully. *(pause)* Put the gift back into the bag and stand up.

Turn around and etch your peaceful place into your mind. All the sights. All the sounds. All the smells. And especially, all the love. Remember you can return here anytime you wish. This is your peaceful place, your place of healing, learning and love.

Turn around and press the elevator button. The doors open and you step inside. This time, press the button marked number 5. The doors close. One, beginning to come up now, two, becoming more alert, three, halfway there, four, almost home, five, open your eyes fully awake and feeling great.

**Today's Date** _____

# Funsheet #5

## Visualization #5 – Dissolving Guilt

1) What type of flowers did you pick?  Is there a significance?

_____

2) Picture/Incident that they showed you in the pool.

_____

_____

3) What good came out of the incident?

_____

4) How can/did you grow from the incident

_____

5) Am I not responsible?        Yes _____   No _____

6) Is there more for you to see?     Yes _____   No _____

7) What was the gift given to you inside the shopping bag?

_____

**Comments/other recollections:**

_____

_____

_____

## Dissipating Anger

I hope you were able to get some really good information to clarify your situation. As we continue to work on our "A" and Absolve our emotional body, it's important to remember that you may not have gotten all that you need to clear in one sitting. I strongly urge you to write down everything that happened on your Funsheet, and make sure to note whether there are any more guilts that need to be visited. If there aren't, then by all means move on. Just make sure that you place the appropriate information received on your goal sheet under "emotional cause," or on your house of well-being chart under the appropriate solution, if that is what you got.

If there are more for you to see, then write, "More work to be done here" at the bottom of you Funsheet. Keep track. Every time you do the visualization, write down the date at the top so you know where you are. When you have cleared all that needs to be cleared, write "Done" at the bottom of your Funsheet. In this way, you will be able to go back to any of the information you received on any given date. Sometimes we think that we are clear, and then if we go back to Higher Wisdom to ask and make sure, we find out there is something we may have missed or that one issue was partially but not completely cleared out and needs to be looked at again. You get the idea. Keeping track will make life a lot simpler for you.

At this time, you can either keep doing this visualization until you've finished clearing all your guilt issues before going on or you can prepare for the next one and go back to work on more of your guilt later. Either way is fine just so long as you keep track and know where you're at and where you are going.

Moving along with our "A," it's time for us to absolve some of our anger. My acronym for anger is: Aspiration Not Getting Expected Result. Simply put, when we hope or aspire to have a situation go one way, and it doesn't turn out the way we expected it to, we become angry. Here is an example:

Your friend says he'll meet you for lunch at noon at your favorite restaurant. You get there on time, but he's not there. You wait and wait. It's now almost 12:30. You know that he is always late, but this time he made a promise to you and you expected him to keep it. As the clock begins to tick away, the steam in your system starts to boil. You head is asking, "Why did I believe him? How could he do such a thing to me? He knows I only have an hour for lunch. " By 12:45, you're seething and you'll probably storm back to work and take it out on the next person that comes into your world. I feel sorry for the poor waitress that has you for a customer after you've been kept waiting that long. Now, in this example you "aspired," or wished to have lunch with a friend and you "expected" to eat with him in a timely fashion so that you could get back to work.

This type of anger is easy to pick out and it happens all the time. What I want you to get from these examples, is that it is not what really happened in your world that is bothering you, so much as what you "expected" to happen in your world. When life doesn't turn out the way we expect it to, we become angry. But let's look a little closer: Are we really angry with him or angry with ourselves?

In the above example, after we complained about the other person, usually the next thought was, "How could I let that happen to me? I should have known better. " In essence, we are never truly angry with the other person, we are always angry with ourselves. Then we feed all that negative emotion and spit it out onto somebody else - sometimes onto an innocent bystander, who just happens to be in the wrong place at the wrong time.

In the same example of the lunch date, if your friend is usually on time, you expect his action to be punctual. Therefore, when presented with the possibility of him being late, your assessment might be, "Gee, he must be stuck in traffic, or maybe he got into an accident. " With that assessment you wouldn't feel angry, you'd feel worry or concern. But when you make the assessment, "He's always late but this time he promised me he'd be on time," you definitely experience anger. Why? Because you expected him to keep his promise, no matter what his former behaviors were. This is like a double whammy. Not only was he inconsiderate of your time but his word doesn't count for anything either: a) you expected him to keep his promise and, b) you expected him to go against his nature. Now, think about this for a minute. It's not even rational. That's like asking an alcoholic to stop drinking and believing him when he tells you what you want to hear.

Here's another example. Your boss is going to make an announcement about a new supervisory position in your department. You have had the best evaluations of everyone. You are the most qualified for the job and were told by everyone that you were a shoe-in. Five minutes before the announcement, a new guy walks into the office and the boss introduces him as the new person in charge of the department. You try to cover up your feelings of disappointment but it is much more than that. Again, your brain is asking, "How could my boss do this to me? " while your mouth is saying "congratulations" to the newcomer.

Remember, in both of these examples, the anger did not come from what they did but what you said in your head about what they did. When you finally said the words in your head, "How could I be so stupid? I should never have trusted him," you blamed yourself and that is what is at the root of all anger—self blame. To put it in a nutshell, anger has two parts: 1) the set up, which is expectation, and 2) the let down, which is self-blame. We actually construct the whole scenario in our head.

So how do we get out of anger without killing someone or losing control? I've said it before. Take a few deep breaths and try to look at the situation from another angle. Try to find the good in everything. If my friend weren't late for our lunch date, I never would have had time to read a magazine, or to watch the blue sky, or to be alone with myself. Whatever.

I remember one of the best days of my life was being stuck in the St.

Louis airport for over thirteen hours. I had been flying standby from Tampa on my way to visit a friend in LA. When I arrived in St. Louis about 8:30 a. m. central time, my connecting flight to Los Angeles had a mechanical problem and they had to cancel the flight. When the next flight became available a couple of hours later, there was no room to accommodate the passengers that were already booked on that flight plus all the stranded passengers left over from the flight before. It was a nightmare. The people were screaming, demanding their money back and generally giving the agents a very hard time.

Three other stranded stand-by passengers and myself started talking. One was going to be in a bridal party the next day and the other had urgent business in LA. It was very stressful for all of us. We kept moving from gate to gate every couple of hours trying to get onto any flight to LA. At one point we decided to go to dinner. In an effort to ease tension, we came up with a new version of Monopoly. We called it Airline Monopoly. Roll the dice and pick a card. Oops, ticket agent made a mistake. You have a child's seat. Sit in the lap of the person next to you. Ah ha in-flight telephone forgets to disconnect: fine, pay $500. Oh ho! Favorable tailwinds - arrive on time, advance to Go, and collect $200. Flight attendant drops soup in your lap, automatic pilot veers flight off course, go back nine spaces. The jokes kept coming and we found ourselves laughing through all our frustration. By nine o'clock we were finally able to get onto a flight to Orange County. Once we arrived there, we shared the cost of a rental car and drove back to LA. I never heard or saw from those people again but I'll remember that happy day for as long as I live.

As I said before, find the good in the situation or make it up. It doesn't serve us to stay angry. Anger that is not resolved turns to rage, and rage turns into something that is red, inflamed, swollen, or painful in the body, like arthritis, carpal tunnel, ulcers, skin blotches, teeth and gum diseases, male dysfunction, female problems and infections of all sorts.

After you've found the good in a bad situation, it's time to turn to forgiveness. We don't forgive others because it helps them; we do it because it releases all the negative energy we've been storing up within ourselves. Forgiveness is something we do heal us. When we let it go, we feel lighter and are better able to cope with the situation at hand. We can't make good judgments or decisions when we are angry. We can't find solutions to any problems when we are angry or in any negative emotion for that matter. Find your peace and that peace will set you free. Free from pain, free from disease, and free from disappointment born of expectation.

Okay. Let's do it! Pop in CD #2, Track #2 *Dissipating Anger* and get ready to let it go. Then fill out your corresponding Funsheet when you've finished and continue reading. I hope you're feeling calmer. My personal students have told me that when they finally let go of their anger, it was as though a cool breeze swept into their heart and created a strong sense of peace.

Don't forget to write down everything that you experienced in as much detail as you can recall. Also, move any of the pertinent information to either your *Goal Sheet* or your *House of Well-Being Chart*. These notes will be immensely helpful to you as a reminder of how light it feels to finally let go.

## Visualization # 6 – *Dissipating Anger*

Get into a very comfortable position and place the tips of your thumb and index fingers of each hand together to form a circle and make the OK sign. Keeping your fingers in the OK position, turn your hands palm side up. Now rest them either on top or along side your legs. Now close your eyes. Begin to drift with the music as it gently flows over you.

Imagine a large blackboard in front of you. Inhale deeply. Hold the breath *(for the count of 7).* Exhale slowly. See the numbers 3, 3, 3. Inhale.

Hold the breath (*for the count of 7*). Exhale. See the numbers 2, 2, 2. Inhale. Hold the breath (*for the count of 7*). Exhale. See the numbers 1, 1, 1

You are standing in the hallway of a very posh hotel on the 10th floor in front of the elevator. Press the call button. Watch the elevator doors now open and step inside. Press the button that is one below the 1st floor. It is marked PP. The doors begin to close. Now watch the lights above the door as you begin to descend. 10, going down, 9, further down, 8, quiet, 7, relaxed, 6, tranquil, 5, silent, 4, serene, 3, calm, 2, harmonious, 1, love, PP, peaceful place.

The doors open up onto the most breathtaking peaceful place you can possibly imagine. The sun is bright. The sky is clear blue. There are several giant puffy white clouds floating overhead. The air smells so sweet and the dew is so fresh. There are birds in the trees and you can hear them sing merrily.

In front of you is a yellow brick path. It is called the Road to Clarity. To the left of the path is a body of water. It is your favorite body of water and there is a cool mist in the air. It caresses your face.

To the right of the yellow brick path is a garden full of your favorite flowers. Bend down and smell the flowers. They are colorful and smell so wonderful. Ask the bushes if you may pick a flower. Watch for them to giggle. It is your sign that it's okay. Now pick two of the most beautiful blooms. Thank the bush for its gift. Now start walking up the yellow brick path.

At about 15 paces or so, you will come to three directional signs. One points to the left; one straight ahead and one to the right. Take the path to the right - the one marked Cottage. Continue walking up the yellow brick path. Enjoy the beautiful landscaping and trees on each side of the path, the fresh clean air and the joyful sound of the birds singing.

At about 20 paces you will come to a picturesque cottage. It has a shingle roof and is painted your favorite colors. (*pause*) Walk up to the front door and ring the bell. Opening the door is one of your healing angels. He or she motions for you to come inside. The room is warm from the burning logs in the fireplace. Another angel is sitting near the hearth on a pillow on the floor. Greet your angels and then hand each of them a flower. *(pause)* Introduce yourself and ask him/her to speak or write his/her name on the tablet that he/she is holding. *(pause 15 seconds)* Now sit down and get comfortable.

This is a very special cottage. It is a place where you can come to relax, enjoy the fire's glow on a chilly day and be alone with your thoughts. It is a place to read and to rid yourself of any negative emotions.

One of your angels gets up and goes to the bookcase alongside the fireplace and pulls down your family album. The cover says, *This is Your Life*. It is a most remarkable book. Not only does it contain pictures, letters, and documents, it also can show holographic images that speak, sing and make music or special sounds. It can even convey feelings without words or pictures. It actually communicates to you in any form that is easy for you to understand.

Ask your angels to turn to the page that marks the incident that sparked your anger resulting in your present state of health. *(pause 30 seconds)*

Say, "Thank you for showing that to me. May I please see the heart and intent of that person at that time?" *(pause 15 seconds)*

Tear the page out of the book and toss it into the fire. *(pause)* Watch it slowly burn and take your anger with it. The anger that you have been experiencing begins to die down. *(pause)* As the smoke rises up into the chimney, your anger is swept away with it, leaving only ashes behind. *(pause)* It is cooled now and the fire is completely out.

Turn back to your angels and ask them if there is more anger for you to clear out of the book. *(pause)* If yes, tell them that you will come back another time *(pause)*. Close the book for now and place it back onto the shelf.

Your angels hand you an envelope and ask you to open it later when you are alone. Put it into your pocket and thank them for all their help and support. *(pause)* This time leave by the back door. Alongside the back porch is a prayer garden. Find a comfortable spot either to sit or kneel.

Pray, "Beloved Creator, I thank you for sending your angels to help me relinquish my anger. I now see that everything was in Your Divine Order and that there is no longer any reason for me to hold onto this."

Visualize a soft pink bubble around the other person or people involved. Then say, "I surround that person and myself in your pink light of love and thereby dissolve all negativity. I forgive them and most of all I forgive myself for holding onto this anger for so long. I now relinquish my anger to You, that it may be dissipated forever." So be it and so it is, amen.

Feel the warmth and the love of your Creator as it permeates your entire being right down to your inner core - your soul. *(pause)* Take a deep breath and blow the soft pink bubble away from you. *(pause)*

The other person dissolves into the distance still surrounded by pink light and you suddenly feel so much lighter, so much happier.

It's time for you to leave your garden. Step around to the front of the cottage and back up the yellow brick path toward the elevator. *(pause)* At the left side of the elevator door is a small bench. Go and sit on it. *(pause)* Now reach into your pocket and open the envelope. Read it carefully. *(pause 15 seconds)* Close it and put it back into your pocket.

Turn around once more and etch your peaceful place into your mind - all the sights, all the sounds, all the smells and especially, all the Love. Remember, you can return here anytime you wish. This is your Peaceful Place, your place of healing, learning and love.

Turn around and press the elevator call button. The doors open and you step inside. This time, press the button marked number 5. The doors close. One, beginning to come up now, two, becoming more alert, three, halfway there, four, almost home, five, open your eyes fully awake and feeling great.

**Today's Date** _____

# Funsheet #6

## Visualization #6 – Dissipating Anger

1) What type of flowers did you pick?   Is there a significance?

_____

2) Did you get the names of your angels when you greeted them at the door?   If so, what were they?

_____

3) What was the incident/people they showed you from the book of your life?

_____

_____

_____

4) Is there more for you to see?    Yes _____    No _____

5) What was in the envelope?

_____

**Comments/other recollections:**

_____

_____

## Overcoming Fear

Moving along with our Letter "A", I guess the hardest lesson that each of us has to learn when we come down to earth is to overcome our fears. Let's look at this situation sensibly. The word fear has also been referred to as: False Evidence Appearing Real. It means that fear is an illusion. It is not an emotion that is based in the here and now. It is based on a possible outcome in the future. It only happens some of the time and if it does, it's never as bad as we imagined it to be.

Fear is created from the energy of our own mind when our thoughts are saying, "What if, what if, what if. " "What if this happens? " or "What if that doesn't happen? " or "How will I ever do this? " When we go round and round and round in our head with these types of scenarios, the body begins to respond. Remember, the body follows the mind. A signal is then sent from our thoughts directly to our heart chakra, which not only controls the heart but the lungs and the bronchi as well.

Have you ever heard the expression, "paralyzed by fear? " That is exactly what happens to us if we let those thoughts go unchecked. Sometimes it gets so bad we can't even breathe. We go into shortness of breath and pass out or have a heart attack. You might say that although the heart chakra is supposed to be open to the giving and receiving of love, fear is the emotion that can shut it down.

What is so sad about living a life in fear is that one winds up living in avoidance of this or that and making decisions based on what is comfortable. You know, don't rock the boat and things like that. Unless we become fearless, we can never truly experience everything that life has to offer. Now, I'm not talking about jumping out of airplanes at two thousand feet, but I do mean taking chances on love and creating grander visions of whom we might be.

Fear not only destroys our ability to fully participate in life, it also keeps us playing small. You'll never write the great American novel, build the greatest invention, start a new business, or sing the highest note, if you don't learn to walk through your fear. What strikes me is that so many of us continue to live our lives as though some imaginary being out there is just waiting to pounce on us, take our belongings, or destroy us. That is simply not true. It's not Universal Truth and it certainly is not my truth.

Fear is simply an experience that is letting us know that we are not connected to our Creator. If I have not said this before, I'll say it again: Co-Creative beings cannot be sick, cannot be broke, cannot be dead, and cannot be alone. These are illusionary experiences or challenges that we attract to us. They are not meant to be a permanent condition. They come so we can learn. They didn't come to "stay", they came to "pass". They do not stay unless we harbor them. I can already hear you protesting: "Not me. I don't harbor fear. I'm not afraid of anything. "

Oh, really! Have you ever noticed how many euphemisms we have in the English language for fear? Let's see, there's "I'm worried. I'm concerned. I really dread. It makes me tremble. It's absolutely disquieting. " Shall I go on? How about "I've had second thoughts or misgivings, I'm not sure. It makes me shake. I shudder to think. I'm just shy. I'm a little nervous. I've got butterflies in my stomach. Got cold feet. I've got this sinking feeling. You know, I don't trust so and so. " Does this sound familiar to you? Actually my synonym finder has no less than seventy-nine euphemisms for fear. No wonder no one can recognize it. We have too many words to cover it up!

Not only do we have words to cover it up, we have another whole basket of different types of fears. Let's see, there is Fear of Lack. That's not having enough of something or being afraid that you can't ever get enough of something. Then there's Fear of Death. Well, that's obvious. Fear of Love, and Fear of not doing the right thing (that, by the way, is guilt.) Then there's Fear of Commitment. The guys taught us gals about that one. And even Fear of Accomplishment and Success. Boy, have I been staring at that one.

Yeah, that's right, even me. I know you find that hard to believe, but no one on the planet, not even me, I don't care who he or she may claim to be, does not experience some type of fear. It's part of the human experience. The difference is that those of us who are living life at a more masterful level can move through it more easily and not allow it to destroy the quality of our lives or the health of our bodies. How do we do that? By keeping our thoughts, words and actions in check.

Whenever we listen to our fearful thoughts, then speak them aloud around the water cooler, we breathe life into them and make them real. Remember thought / word / action? Unwitting statements like, "You know, there's a rumor that the new boss is going to make a big announcement on Monday. " Now that might not sound fearful, but the thought behind that statement is, "Am I going to have a job on Monday after cutbacks? " Or how about this one: "I don't like this pain in my leg. " Now the thought and the meaning behind that one is, "I've not been taking care of my body and I don't know what awful thing is going to happen to me. "

Remember, when I speak Creator speaks, and when you speak Creator speaks, and when Creator speaks, SO IT IS. With that understanding, you can see that WE are the architects of all the fearful challenges that come into our life.

Now there are some who would say, "That can't be true. What if a thief holds a gun to your head? You couldn't possibly have had anything to do with that. " Oh, you think so? By now you must have surmised that the thief would not have come into your path if, on some level, your fear hadn't called him forth. I know that's difficult to swallow but think of it this way. Nothing in the Universe happens by accident. Remember, there are no victims and no villains. Everything is in Divine Right Order. "

A great teacher known as Abraham explains it this way. Imagine a large round table top with a million holes in it. Inside each tiny hole there is a light shining. The whole tabletop is a massive light board. The lights twinkle in different colors. And then the colors change according to the frequency they are emitting. WE are those lights. When we are emitting love for instance, we are blinking, say, on a pink frequency. All the other pink lights on the board are then attracted to us, blink back, and answer our call. These are people who come into our world to help us experience love. If we are in fear, however, we're probably blinking say, on red, and wind up attracting other red lights. These are people who show up in our world to help us experience fear. They don't have to be murderers or thieves, they could simply be gregarious or manipulative people, or people who are in power, the police, the IRS, or even your friendly doctor, who just happens to have some bad news for you. They could also be those cold types that speak without thinking and hurt our feelings. Or it can be your boss who doesn't give you a promotion or a raise when we really deserve it.

You see, the people that answer the call are just responding to what we sent out. If we don't think we are good enough, then a dozen people will surely show up in our to prove us right. Haven't you ever noticed how each of us is always right in our own life? That is how the Universe works. Whatever we send out we get back.

So what's the point of all of this? Well it's Self Love. Now, I'm not talking about looking in the mirror and being narcissic or anything like that. What I'm saying is that if we want to live a happy, healthy and productive life, we must start by loving ourselves first. Loving and nurturing self is paramount to keeping our soul and our health intact. Living in fear is not trusting that we are Co-Creative partners with Our Creator and that together we can solve any problem. It is not trusting that the solution will show up in time and that all is well in our world and in the world around us. When we remain in fear, we literally cut ourselves off from what some call "the stream of wellness," which is Love, Creator, God/Goddess, the Universe, ALL THAT IS. We are love. Anything that pulls us away from who we are is bound to cause us hardship and illness. When we are not connected to the source of our being, we are not loving self. When we are not loving self, we have little or no love to give to another.

The biblical directive was to "Love thy neighbor AS thyself. " Not "more than," not "less than," and not "instead of," but "AS. " How can we ask for love from another, when we are not willing to give it to ourselves? What kind of relationship results from that? I'll tell you what kind, a co-dependent relationship. A relationship in which each one is depending on the other for self-esteem, nurturing and respect. Ever wonder why the divorce rate is so high? These relationships are doomed to fail because no one can bear the weight of providing all of that to another person 24/7 and that, my friend, is why we are so unhappy. We feel inadequate.

Please remember to be good to yourself first. When you feel that warmth in your chest and know that everything is right within you, spread that joyous feeling around and watch it come back to you tenfold. Silence the little voice in your head that creates worry and fear by saying, "Mind be still and know that I am love. " I promise you, you'll never have one day of sickness if you do.

One final word, there is such a thing as caution. Caution is protecting yourself, like looking both ways before you cross the street. Protection is another form of loving self. If you ever find yourself in any relationship in which you feel that you need to be protected from the other party, I beg you, please get out. No one, not parent, child or spouse, is required to stay in any type of abusive relationship, whether that be physical, mental, or especially verbal / emotional abuse. Recognize it for what it is, an opportunity to learn the lesson of "sovereigncy of self," which is independence and protecting yourself first. Send love and light to that other person and cut the cord. Life is to short to stop loving yourself because you feel an obligation to a particular relationship. No one is better than you or more important than you. When you honor self, you honor the Holy Spirit or Creator God / Goddess within.

## An Exercise

Before we do our next visualization, I'd like you to try this short exercise. Take a minute to think about someone in your life that you absolutely love. Now I said love, not lust. That could be anybody. A friend, a relative, an associate, or it could be a very kind person that you barely know, or it could be a spouse or a lover. Now close your eyes, take a very deep breath and exhale. See that person very clearly in front of you. Call forth every detail of his or her face. Also remember the aspects of that person that make you love them: their kindness, their consideration, the way they touch you, the way they speak to you. Now hold the thought. Experience the feeling that goes with this thought. Surround yourself with this wondrous feeling. Now file it in your memory under "this is what my love feels like. " Now open your eyes.

The reason that I had you do this is because I want you to be able to instantly recognize feelings of love. This is the feeling that you shall experience while communicating with your angels. If for any reason, you do not feel this, immediately ask, "Are you from the light? " They should smile and answer quickly. If there is no answer, or it just doesn't feel right, just see yourself encapsulated in a white diamond and say, "I am of the light, I am of the light, I am of the light. I choose not to communicate with you. Be gone!" That will easily take care of it because they must obey us. That is Universal Law. It's only on rare occasions we are tested so that we know who and who not to talk to. This is called the "lesson of discernment. " It's no big deal. No harm can come to you if you did speak with lower thought forms. You simply wouldn't get the best answers. They are not evil or bad, and they have absolutely no power over you. They are simply around to confuse us to teach us the lesson of discernment. That's their job. To help us understand how powerful we truly are.

How to avoid this? Simple, my angels have given us an insurance policy. They suggest that you say a prayer of protection before you do any type of communicating. The one they gave me is on Page 24 of your Funbook: "Beloved Creator, I ask for the white light of protection, over me, under me, round and about, in and out, and in all the nooks and crannies. I ask for a clear transmission to the angels of light, and I ask the Masters of the Light Brotherhood to intensify this light, honor, bless and keep me. So be it and so it is. Amen. "

You might experience a tingling sensation. It's very common. Just enjoy the feeling. Now, you can use this prayer or make up one of your own. Whichever you choose is fine. Just visualize yourself completely surrounded by a silvery white color as you say it. You could see yourself in the middle of a silver white ball, or a pyramid or white diamond. It is your intent that moves the energy in the Universe. Use whichever picture feels most comfortable to you.

Okay. We've taken a good look at the why and how of fear, and now its your turn to start shedding some light on your own by doing your Overcoming Fear visualization. Remember all you have to do with a particular fear is to shed light on it, then dissipate it back to the Universe. Then that one is gone forever and can no longer injure your body. Most of my students tell me that once they have completed this visualization, they feel so much lighter. Like a huge burden has been lifted. You'll be fine. As I said before, intention moves the energy of the Universe. Here and now, it is my intention to surround you in my love and place you under the protection of the Masters of the Family of Light. You are in good hands. Like Nike advises, "Just do it. " When you're done, fill out your Funsheet for this visualization. Make any notes in your Goal Sheet or House of Well Being Chart and come back.

Please remember three things:
a) Fear is at the root of all your negative energy and therefore is holding your illnesses and challenges in place.

b) You are not alone.   There will be angels to guard and protect you and

c) My love surrounds you always.

Go for it!  Pop in CD #2, Track #3 – or record the following script

## Visualization # 7 – *Overcoming Fear*

Get into a very comfortable position and place the tips of your thumb and index fingers of each hand together to form a circle and make the okay sign.  Keeping your fingers in the okay position, turn your hands palm side up.  Now rest them either on top of or along side your legs.  Close your eyes. Begin to drift with the music as it gently flows over you.

Imagine a large blackboard in front of you.   Inhale deeply.   Hold the breath *(for the count of 7)*.   Exhale slowly.   See the numbers 3, 3, 3.   Inhale. Hold the breath *(for the count of 7)*. Exhale.   See the numbers 2, 2, 2.   Inhale. Hold the breath *(for the count of 7)*.   Exhale.   See the numbers 1, 1, 1

You are standing in the hallway of a very posh hotel on the 10th floor in front of the elevator.  Press the call button.   Watch the elevator doors open and step inside.  Press the button that is one below the 1st floor.  It is marked PP.  The doors begin to close.  Now watch the lights above the door as you begin to descend.  10, going down, 9, further down, 8, quiet, 7, relaxed, 6, tranquil, 5, silent, 4, serene, 3, calm, 2, harmonious, 1, love, PP, peaceful place.

The doors open up onto the most breathtaking peaceful place you can possibly imagine.  The sun is bright.  The sky is blue.  There are several giant puffy white clouds floating overhead.  The air smells so sweet and the dew is so fresh.  There are birds in the trees and you can hear them singing merrily.

In front of you is a yellow brick path.  It is called the Road to Clarity. To the left of the path is a body of water.  It is your favorite body of water and there is a cool mist in the air and it caresses your face.

To the right of the yellow brick path is a garden full of your favorite flowers.  Bend down and smell the flowers.  They are colorful and smell so wonderful.  Ask the bushes if you may pick a flower.  Watch them giggle.  It

137

is your sign that it's okay. Now pick two of the most beautiful blooms. Thank the bush for its gift. Now start walking up the yellow brick path.

At about 15 paces you will come to three directional signs. One points to the left. one straight ahead and one to the right. Take the path to the right. The one marked Theatre. Continue walking and observe the beautiful landscaping and trees on each side of the path. At about 10 paces you will come to a silvery white gate. Waiting at the gate are two healing angels, one male and one female. They open the gate for you. Greet your angels, introduce yourself and ask him or him to speak his/her name or write it on the tablet that he/she is holding. *(pause)* Hand each of them a flower. They thank you and motion you to follow them up to the front row and take the center seat. One angel sits on your left and one on your right.

This is a very unique theatre. It can show you slide pictures. It can create special music or sounds to communicate to you. It can even reach you through your feelings or your sense of smell. Your angels are about to help you see either through pictures, words, music or feelings that which you need to know to help accelerate your healing process. Take a deep breath and as you exhale, begin to focus your attention on the screen. *(pause)* You are completely relaxed and ready to experience what they are trying to show you. Now turn to your angels and ask them to show you your first worry. *(pause 15 seconds)*

Hold that picture, sound or sense and then say, "Thank you for showing that to me but it is no longer part of my reality". *(pause)* Now surround the picture, sound or feeling in a violet light and say, "I transmute this energy into Love". *(pause)* Watch it dissolve into tiny violet particles of light. The screen fades to black.

"Angels, show me my next worry." *(pause 15 seconds)* "That, too, is no longer part of my reality. I surround this anxiety with the violet light and transmute it into Love". *(pause)* Now watch this dissolve into tiny violet particles of light. The screen again turns to black.

"Show me my last worry." *(pause 15 seconds)*   "This is also no longer part of my reality.  I surround this anxiety with the violet light and transmute it back into Love. *(pause)*   It. Too, dissolves into tiny violet particles of light. Your screen again fades to black.

Turn to your angels and ask them if there is anything else you have to see.  If they say yes, tell them you will come back next time. *(pause)*   Thank your angels for their assistance. *(pause 15 seconds)*

Your angels begin to rise from their seats.  Follow them back to the gate and say your farewells.  You may wish to give them a hug. *(pause)*  Wave goodbye and start walking back up the yellow brick path towards the elevator door.

Now once more, turn around and etch your peaceful place into your mind - all the sights, sounds, smells, and especially all the Love.  Remember you can return here anytime you wish.  This is your peaceful place - your place of healing, learning and love.

Turn around and press the elevator button.  The doors open and you step inside.  This time, press the button marked number 5.  The doors close. One, beginning to come up now, two, becoming more alert, three, halfway there, four, almost home, five, open your eyes fully awake and feeling great.

**Today's Date** _____

# Funsheet #7

## Visualization #7 – Overcoming Fear

**1)  What type of flowers did you pick?   Is there a significance?**

_____

2)  **First Worry?**

_____

_____

3)  **Second Worry?**

_____

_____

4)  **Third Worry?**

_____

_____

**5)  Are there any more for you to see?     Yes _____     No _____**

## Comments/recollections:

_____

_____

_____

_____

_____

# Chapter 9

## Request Loving Angels both Human and Spiritual

## Letter "L"

### "L" – Line Up Physical Assistance

If no one has ever said this to you before, let me be the first. I acknowledge your bravery. I know it took courage to look at your fears, but think of it this way: they're gone now and can no longer rule you. Again, I urge you to write down as much as you can remember in the "Comments" section of your Funsheet. I must admit that I have a special reason to keep you writing. When you journal, you are adding the directive of "word" to your thoughts. Remember thought, word and action? By writing down your experiences and the results, your negative energy clears twice as fast and you heal even faster.

You might be thinking "How could communicating with my angels be under the category of physical assistance and not under spiritual assistance? Actually, it belongs under both categories, A and L, "A" for absolving and connecting with your spiritual body and "L" for lining up physical assistance. When you are "in communion" with your angels/guides, you will be able to ask any question you wish, including, "Who would the best person be to help me with this situation? " An answer to that question is indeed "physical assistance coming from a spiritual source".

If you ask, you can have a special angel come to you that is knowledgeable in natural medicines. Mine was Li Sung an ancient Chinese herbalist and spiritual teacher. He taught me the importance of herbs and how to dose them for myself correctly. He encouraged me to purchase books from present-day authors and to study whenever possible. I took his advice and always keep an herbal reference book on hand.

Okay. The moment you've been waiting for has finally arrived. You have been diligently working on your letter A, Absolving your emotional bodies since Chapter 7. At last you have an opportunity to move into communicating with your own personal Angel. This one has been especially assigned to you for this experience. But before we begin, let's take a little review about angels.

The word angel is usually inferred to mean "messenger," but they also perform many other tasks. They guide. They teach. They offer comfort and give wisdom. They warn us and protect us from danger. They help tune our bodies to cope with what used to be three-dimensional living and is now multi or fifth dimensional living. They inspire us and can even help re-balance our aura, if we so desire or request it. For these reasons, they have been called by many names such as "guides, muses, guardians, or master teachers. " Basically any spiritual entity in the etheric realms (heaven) that chooses to do service is an angel.

They also have a rank or standing among themselves. This ranking is not determined by chronological age, but rather by the number of experiences they have had and how much wisdom they have garnered. The more they have learned, they higher they ascend. The youngest or least experienced are usually depicted as naked babies or cherubs. This grouping is called the cherubim. I doubt seriously that they actually look like that, but the childlike image denotes a fledgling angel just getting its wings.

The next up the ladder are the Seraphim, who are usually painted as adults or teenagers and appear to be more mature and wise. And then of course, there are the Elohim, or the master teachers, which are commonly referred to as archangels. Although the number of archangels in the universe is constant at 144,000, there are only about six that made headlines in the bible. Some of these unknowns may actually be here on earth at this time, to assist with the elevation of the spirituality of the planet. These wondrous teachers can be found in every spiritual tradition and are usually referred to in the many holy books written throughout history. Sometimes we refer to them as prophets or saints and they have also been called the star seeds or the creator gods. They were the highest light frequency beings that evolved when God split and individuated to create the universe. Basically, angels are light beings, who may or may not have visited the planet and have volunteered to do service.

Angels live in many realms. Some are close to earth, but there are many in other star systems, such as Sirrius, the Pleiades, and Orion. Then there is Illiac, Maladek, and Solonika. Unfortunately I can't pinpoint all of these realms on a star map. As a matter of fact, some of them may not even be physical places. They may simply be planes of consciousness. All I know is that these places do exist and that you and I probably came from somewhere out there. I guess that sort of makes all of us extra-terrestrials. Hey! Beam me up, Scotty! I don't want to be late for dinner. Oh well, back to the third moving into fifth dimension.

My master teachers tell me that we all have at least one angel. One will stay with us throughout our lifetime while we're here on earth, but there are many others that will come and go, depending on our needs. You've probably heard the saying, "When the student is ready, the teacher will appear. " Well, then, don't be surprised if, during your lifetime, your angels change. As a matter of fact, if you simply ask that whatever angel is best able to help you with a particular problem or need come forward, a different one may appear at each new request. In that way, you can build a team of angels to help you with the different areas of your life. For instance, when I am in financial trouble, I call upon Sylvestri. He is my angel of finance. When I'm

No Such Thing as Incurable

having relationship problems, I call upon my Group from the Pleiades.  I have even called upon Arabella, my angel of music, to help me with choosing the musical keys for the visualizations in this book.

Each of your angels has a personality all his or her own, just like people here.  Some are funny, some are soft spoken, and some are loud and strong.  Some are even downright tough.  Which brings me to the question: "Can people who were in your family and have made their transition become one of your angel team? " The answer is "yes. " Anyone who has been on the earth and wants to do service for those they left behind is automatically available, which is practically everyone.  So you can call up your grandmother or your favorite uncle in spirit for help and don't be surprised if they act the same way they did when they were here, even grouchy!

You can also ask for a particular angel, like a great prophet that you admire.  He or she will come when your thoughts are read.  However, in order for you to telepathically communicate with him or her, you must be able to reach his or her frequency.  They can come down halfway, but we must go up the other half.  To reach them, we must sincerely desire to communicate, have purity of intent to live masterfully and continually practice opening up our throat and third eye chakras.  That takes a few prayers, a little time, practice and patience.  There's no way that I know of to measure where you are or whom you can reach.  It is simply a matter of trial and error, so please don't give up.

There's not much more that I can say here about angels except to talk about them is also to talk about love.  Love that is given unconditionally is the most precious gift anyone of us can give or receive.  It is that safe feeling that spurs us to accept others as they are without judgment and without wanting or asking them to change.   Angels are within the light and love of Creator / God / Goddess / All That Is and love us for who we are and honor us just for coming here.

My master teachers, whom I refer to as the Masters of the Family of

146

Light say that they are "ever ready to be of service, and wish to extend an invitation to you to join one of them at the top of the mountain. " Guys, the red carpet is waiting.

Pop in CD #2 – Track #4 – *Talking with your Angel,* or record the following script for your personal mediation and have a nice visit. Afterwards, fill in your Funsheet.

## Visualization #8 – *Talking with your Angel*

Get into a very comfortable position and place the tips of your thumb and index fingers of each hand together to form a circle and make the okay sign. Keeping your fingers in the okay position, turn your hands palm side up. Now rest them either on top or along side your legs. Now close your eyes. Begin to drift with the music as it gently flows over you.

Imagine a large blackboard in front of you. Now inhale deeply. Hold the breath *(for the count of 7).* Exhale slowly. See the numbers 3, 3, 3. Inhale. Hold the breath *(for the count of 7).* Exhale. See the numbers 2, 2, 2. Inhale. Hold the breath *(for the count of 7).* Exhale. See the numbers 1, 1, 1

You are standing in the hallway of a very posh hotel on the 10th floor in front of the elevator. Press the call button. Watch the elevator doors now open and step inside. Press the button that is one below the 1st floor. It is marked PP. The doors begin to close. Now watch the lights above the door as you begin to descend. 10, going down, 9, further down, 8, quiet, 7, relaxed, 6, tranquil, 5, silent, 4, serene, 3, calm, 2, harmonious, 1, love, PP, peaceful place.

The doors open up onto the most breathtaking peaceful place you can possibly imagine. The sun is bright. The sky is blue. There are several giant puffy white clouds floating overhead. The air smells so sweet and the dew so fresh. There are birds are singing in the trees.

In front of you is a yellow brick path. It is called the Road to Clarity. To the left of the path is a body of water. It is your favorite body of water

To the right of the yellow brick path is a beautifully landscaped flower garden. It is full of your favorite flowers. Go over smell the flowers. They are bright, vibrant and pungent. Ask them if you may pick a bloom. When they move and giggle, it's your sign that it's okay. Pick the most radiant bloom. Thank the flowers for their gift. Turn around and start walking up the yellow brick path.

At about 15 paces the road forks into three paths. One path goes to the left, one to the right and one straight ahead. Each path has a directional sign. Take the left fork, the one marked "Mountain."

Continue up the left path and observe the beautiful trees and plants that create this spectacular nature walk. *(pause)* At about 20 paces, you will see a beautiful silver white bubble waiting for you at the foot of the mountain. Step into the bubble. This beautiful silver white light permeates every cell of your being, over you, under you, around and about, in an out and in all your nooks and crannies. It is here to uplift you and to protect you on your journey up the mountain. Your silver white light bubble has become entirely absorbed into your being. *(pause)*

Turn your attention to your feet and you will see this beautiful sparkling clear staircase. It winds as far as the eye can see around the mountain all the way to the top. Take hold of the handrail and begin to climb effortlessly. The steps are close together and there is no strain at all.

As you start your ascent, you can see the squirrels and rabbits scurrying around and the tall pines bending in the breeze. In between the shrubs you can even get a glimpse of a white tail deer. You keep climbing and the air becomes thick with the sweet smell of fresh rain.

You are on the far side of the mountain now and you see this beautiful magnificent waterfall. It cascades down the side of the mountain into a small pool below. You can hear the splashing of the water as it hits the pool.

Your eyes turn away from the waterfall to a series of carved tablets on the side of the mountain. They were placed there by an ancient civilization just for you to discover.  Take a good look.  They have a picture or message just for you.  *(pause 10 seconds)*

Only a few more feet and you will be at the top of the mountain.  You now step onto this sacred ground.  In front of you is a large tree shading a picnic area.  There waiting for you under the tree is one of your healing angels. Go over and greet your angel.  Introduce yourself and ask him/her to speak his/her name or to write it on the tablet he/she is holding.  *(pause 10 seconds)*

Hand your angel your flower.  He or she also has a gift for you.  This gift has great significance for you at this time.  Allow your angel to explain and continue in conversation as you wish.  Enjoy your visit. *(pause 2 minutes)*

It's time to go home now.  Your angel walks with you to the staircase.  He/she takes you by the hand.  The wings open wide and he/she gently lifts you right back to the foot of the mountain.  *(pause)*  You both touch down safely and securely.

Thank your angel for taking the time to be with you today.  *(pause)* Say your farewells. *(pause)* Turn and start back up the yellow brick path.

You are now in front of the elevator door.  Turn around once more. See you angel in the distance. Know that this is your peaceful place. You can come back here anytime you wish to visit your angels to receive all the wisdom, all the love and all the healing that you desire.  Press the elevator call button.  The doors open.  Step inside and press the number five.  One, beginning to come up now, two, becoming more alert, three, halfway there, four, almost home, five, open your eyes fully awake and feeling great.

Today's Date _____

# Funsheet #8

## Visualization #8 – Talking with your Angel

1)   What type of flowers did you pick?   Is there a significance?

_____

2)   What was on the carved tablets on the side of the mountain?

_____

_____

_____

3)   What did you and your angel talk about?

_____

_____

_____

_____

_____

_____

**Comments/recollections:**

_____

_____

_____

_____

I hope you had a great chat. Did you receive information to help line up physical assistance under your L, or for one of you're A's? In either case, did you jot down all you can remember on your Funsheet for your journal? If not, do it before we continue.

I can't impress upon you enough the need for journaling your experiences. Not only will you be able to look back and see how much you have learned but you will also maintain accurate records for future situations that may come up. It's sort of a report card in the making and it is my sincere hope that you are all getting A+.

# Chapter 10

## Finishing the Letters
## "E" and "D"

### E – Execute Your Program

There once was a very successfully advertising campaign that said, "Just do it. " Why is it so hard for us to write a "to do" list and then follow through? I have no idea but what I do know is that if you don't "do it", you will not achieve any of your healing goals.

If I could only put you up in a fancy hotel, stop all the craziness in your life, feed you high octane food, help you with yoga stretches and hug you for doing such a good job to make your boo boo's go away, I would. Unfortunately I cannot. No healing instrument can. Not even God/Goddess themselves. They can assist, give you encouragement, teachers, tools and supplies but even they cannot do it for you. You are a co-creative being and must create your half. Seems I remember a very old adage here, "God helps those who help themselves". Couldn't have said it better myself.

I have personally seen at least two people who had someone of great notoriety lay hands on them in a public gathering, get up and walk away with a so-called miracle only to have reverted back to their former state of health within days or a few weeks. Although they had been given the gift of grace to know that whatever they had "could" be healed, they were not "ready" to accept the gift because of feelings of unworthiness and/or to release the negative thoughts and emotions that brought the illness into being.

Knowing that a healing may only be temporary is the greatest blow to one who has dedicated his/her life to service of humanity. It's happened to me several times and it broke my heart every time even though I knew that I did my very best. It is truly a humbling experience.

A complete healing can only happen if YOU heal yourself. YOU are the creator of your own illness and in the end YOU are the healer. Your choices, your mindset, your intention, your actions and the intensity of your willingness to participate affect the outcome.

Every miracle drug or natural remedy must be taken. Every body must be purified. Every physical therapy session must be completed. Every mouthful must be considered carefully before chewing and swallowing. Every prayer must be heartfelt. And every negative emotion must be cleared. The quality of the remainder of your life or maybe your life itself is on the line here. This is no time to fool around or cheat on your program. It's time for complete commitment.

If you take nothing else away from these pages, know that you are loved unconditionally whether you pursue your healing journey or not. However, I encourage you to participate fully. I promise that you will find that there are many who will appear seemingly out of nowhere, to assist you, if you simply work the program and ask for guidance. This is time to execute the faith of the mustard seed. Execution is the key that will open the door to a new life for you, if you are courageous enough to walk through its door.

I've extended my hand, given you the tools and sent you love and light to assist you through your journey. The rest is up to YOU. If I must borrow the phrase one more time, please, please JUST DO IT!

# D – Declare thanks to Creator/God/Goddess/All That Is

Every person that I have ever met that came back from a so-called incurable illness has had one common story. They all said that they were grateful for the experience. They had become better people and were now in a position to do something better with their lives or to help others who had encountered the same situation. They had all grown spiritually, mentally, emotionally and physically from their experience and acknowledged their Creator for helping them through it.

For me, looking into the possible face of full-blown cancer made me work my program hard and stimulated me to journal my daily trials. When I finally figured out that I could put at least two sentences together coherently and could use my healing and singing voice to help others, I simply jumped on board. Let me tell you, it's been a roller coaster ride but I wouldn't have changed a thing, except maybe waiting so long to go before the camera. I know it's hard to believe but you might say, I'm a tad camera shy.

When one finally comes to the realization that the debilitating sickness that had been plaguing them so long "came to pass" and not "to stay", one immediately turns to his/her Creator in gratitude. It is simply closure. Your own thank you prayer and resulting warm and confident attitude will push you heads above the rest and assure you that whatever it was that you once had will surely never come back unless your earth bound chapter is done and your soul is truly desiring to leave the planet. Even then, you will know that you are forever whole and will have no fear of moving into the next chapter of your ever-continuing life in angel form. Strange as it may sound, you may even look forward to volunteering to assist humanity from beyond.

# Chapter 11

## Self-Healing Made Easy

We're coming down the home stretch. There's not much more I can say about healing, except to give you a few more guidelines under your "Be Healed" format.

### Guidelines for Healing

**B: Befriend your illness**

a) Don't be afraid of it and don't go to war with it.

b) Immediately say a prayer of gratitude when you first learn of your illness, thanking your Creator for bringing you this great opportunity to learn and grow spiritually, mentally, emotionally and physically.

c) Take responsibility for your own well being.

**E: Eliminate the Pain**

a) Use the power of your mind through visualization whenever possible.

b) Use natural rubs with diluted eucalyptus or inhale lavender essential oil to assist.

**H: Hear the message**

a) Practice listening to your body.

b) Practice listening to your Higher Wisdom.

c) Practice listening to your angels.

**E: Evaluate Your Illness**

a) Make sure you fully understand the name, nature, and ramifications of your illness.

b) Fill out your Funsheets, Goal Sheets, and House of Well Being Chart to create a journal.

c) Follow and check off your "To Do" list until it's completed and you are satisfied with your results.

**A: Absolve (cleanse) All Four Bodies**

a) Clear the physical body of debris and toxins.

b) Clear the mental body of negative thoughts and fears brought up by someone else's negative opinion of what you are doing, by saying: "Mind be still and know that I am love. "

c) Clear the emotional body by forgiving yourself and others, and by removing traces of guilt, anger and fear.

d) Clear the spiritual body by staying connected to your Creator, finding higher truths to believe in and never, ever calling yourself by your disease.

**L: Line Up Physical Assistance**

a) Find a healthy physical surrounding in which to heal.

b) Change the colors of your clothes to help you feel better.

c) Find professional practitioners that know how to integrate western medicine and holistic medicine, giving you the best of both worlds.

d) Increase your nutritional levels.

e) Follow a simple daily exercise routine to strengthen your entire body. Walking is the best choice if you can.

E: Execute Your Program

a) Take immediate action.

b) Fill out your Funsheets and add the information gained to your "to do" list.

c) Check off all your "to do's" as they are completed and stick with your program until you're satisfied with your results.

**D: Declare Thanks to Your Creator**

Everyday, take a moment to thank that Creator / God / Goddess / All That Is, for all you are presently learning and for the opportunity to continue to connect and to grow.

## Tips for your To Do List

It's pretty self-explanatory but I would suggest that you keep it handy to remind yourself to make the necessary entries. Even things that seem trivial could be very important to your healing journey, so please don't discount any information or guidance you may receive.

If you need some more space for more entries, type or design a better one to suit your needs. This one is simply to help you start a detailed program and to make sure you've covered all the bases on one sheet of paper.

# Healing "to do" List

☐ **B** Write a short prayer/affirmation here to befriend your illness.

_____
_____
_____

☐ **E** I have eliminated my pain by

_____

☐ **H** Messages I have received:

1) _____
2) _____
3) _____
4) _____
5) _____
6) _____

☐ **E** I have evaluated my illness by:

1) (diagnosis) _____

2) (severity)_____
3) (time needed to reverse) _____
4) (best choice of treatment) _____
5) (best choice of practitioner) _____
6) (complimentary treatments) _____

☐ **A** I have absolved the following bodies:

Physical by: a) _____
            b) _____
            c) _____

Mental by: a) _____
           b) _____
           c) _____

Emotional by:

    Guilt of _____, _____, _____

    Anger at _____, _____, _____

    Fear of _____, _____, _____

Spiritual by:  a) _____

              b) _____

              c) _____

☐ **L** I have lined up the following physical assistance:

1) _____

2) _____

3) _____

4) _____

5) _____

6) _____

☐ **E** I execute the following program tasks (circle one D = daily, W = weekly, M = monthly):

1) _____ D  W  M

2) _____ D  W  M

3) _____ D  W  M

4) _____ D  W  M

5) _____ D  W  M

6) _____ D  W  M

7) _____ D  W  M

8) _____ D  W  M

9) _____ D  W  M

10) _____ D  W  M

☐ **D** I have declared my thanks to Creator with the following prayer:

_____

_____

_____

_____

# A Final Thought

When I was a teenager, my friends and I would go to Coney Island Beach in Brooklyn, NY every Sunday during the summer. The very last thing we did before taking the subway home was to ride the carousel. The calliope would beckon and, back in those ancient times, the operator would hold out a shaft filled with aluminum rings about the size of a silver dollar. The rings would slide down the shaft for us to catch as our horses rode by. Only one ring was brass. If you caught the brass ring, you got a free ride.

To me, trying to catch the brass ring has become a metaphor for healing our lives. Sometimes we're up, sometimes we're down, and sometimes you get a chance to do it over, only better. The important thing is to stay young at heart, be happy, and enjoy the ride. You see, it's the enjoyment of the journey and living in the now that keeps you healthy.

When I started this book, I had a special intent and finally wrote it into a mission statement, which read: "I wish to enlighten and assist people in the realization that each one of us has a God given natural ability to heal ourselves and that in the highest sense, there is no such thing as incurable. " I truly believe that the ability to self-heal came with our birthday suit the day we arrived on the planet, and that it's for us to individually discover.

It makes me happy to have been of assistance in your self-healing process. I couldn't have done it without the help of a great team at Audiolab, especially Josh Young, who makes me sound a whole lot better on CD than I do in person. Lou Panzer, who wrote the beautiful visualization music and the input and inspiration of the heavenly hosts, the angels, the guides, and Masters of the Family of Light, who assisted me in bringing this information to you.

Surprisingly, this program could not have been completed without you. You see, your light was blinking, and I answered. I thank you for being with me today and I honor you for giving me the opportunity to share my thoughts and experiences with you. I wish you better health, happiness and abundance beyond your wildest imagination. And please remember: No matter how old you are, if you want to stay healthy, remember there is no such thing as incurable and never pass up the chance to "Ride the Carousel…"

# Ride the Carousel

## Words & Music by Annemarie St. Michael
© 2001 *All Rights Reserved*

There was a time, when there was anger in my life.

I passed my prime, and couldn't keep my youthful stride.

Would I ever see my dreams come true and hold my financial stance?

In the end, like my friends, thought I stood no chance.


So I prayed and asked the heavens what to do

Then on the shade, I saw a light beam split in two.

In the dead of night an angel suddenly appeared to me.

He said, "Don't you frown. It will turn around, if you listen carefully. "


CHORUS    Dance like nobody's watching. Laugh like no one else can hear.

Live like there's no tomorrow and love like you have no fear.

Spend like you have a fortune. Play like you know you're well.

If you wanna stay young forever, my friend, *Ride the Carousel*.


Now every day, I look for fun things I can do

And when I pray, I thank the heavens for the news.

I live only in a playful world, 'cause my watch is in the drawer.

I can truly say, in a humble way, I'm younger than before.


CHORUS    Dance like nobody's watching. Laugh like no one else can hear.

Live like there's no tomorrow and love like you have no fear.

Spend like you have a fortune. Play like you know you're well.

If you wanna stay young forever, my friend, *Ride the Carousel*.

# Author's Biography

Annemarie St. Michael; is a living, breathing example of the power of self-healing and serves as inspiration for all who seek well being. She suffered severe rheumatic heart disease as a child then in early adulthood came manic-depression, followed by arthritis, chronic fatigue syndrome then cervical cancer.

For 14 years she has shared her wit and soothing hypnotic voice leading creative visualizations and hypnotic sessions for individuals and large groups as well as assisting the chronically and seriously ill back to health with healing touch.

As an award-winning lyricist/composer/recording artist, St. Michael adds the dimension of beautiful music to her healing lectures. She has discovered that music jump-starts the healing process and uplifts the spirit of those in her audience.

St. Michael, a Registered Hypnotherapist, broadened her scope to encompass her unique brand of creative visualization at the same time adding angelic touch to her list of modalities. She then founded one of the first schools dealing with the various aspects of healing known as the Awakening Circle.

St. Michael has appeared on radio stations across America sharing her knowledge, first hand experiences, love, laughter and beautiful music.

# Bibliography

Balch, James F. & Balch, Phyllis. *Prescription for Nutritional Healing*

Burns, David D. *Feeling Good*

Chopra, Deepak. *Ageless Body, Timeless Mind* and audio tape *Perfect Weight*

Hicks, Ester. *The Law of Attraction: The Basic Teachings of Abraham*

Knight, J.Z. *Voyage to the New World*

Kubler-Ross, Elisabeth. *On Death and Dying*

LaRouche, Loretta. *Life is Short – Wear Your Party Pants*

Merriam-Webster. *Webster's New Collegiate Dictionary*, 1973 Edition

Silva, Jose. *Silva Mind Control*

Sommers, Suzanne. *Eat, Cheat and Melt the Fat Away*

Wallach, Eli and Lan, Ma. *Let's Play Doctor* and audio tape *Dead Doctors Don't Lie*

Walsch, Neale Donald. *Conversations with God, Volume I, Conversations with God Volume II, Conversations with God Volume III*

Weil, Andrew. *8 Weeks to Optimum Health* and *Spontaneous Healing*

Wigmore, Ann. *The Wheatgrass Book: How to Grow and Use Wheatgrass to Maximize Your Health and Vitality*

Wright, Johnathan – *Book of Nutritional Therapy* and *Guide to Healing with Nutrition*

# Free CD Order Form

## *Annemarie St. Michael Visualizations*

     As a special thanks for purchasing this book, I am happy to send you the recorded visualizations that have been scripted in the previous pages. It has been our pleasure to bring you the wisdom and serenity of the angels in these recordings in the hope that you will benefit greatly from your experience of listening and using their messages in your quest for a healthier body and life.

     If you have an uplifting story to share, please write it to me at my website so I can pass it onto others who can also benefit. By the way, you can tell your friends that they will receive the same free offer of eight recorded visualizations should they decide to purchase our book in a store, directly from our headquarters or online at our website.

- - - - - - - - - - - - - - - - - - - - - - - - - - - - - - - - - -

❏ *No Such Thing as Incurable* Visualization Two-CD Set

Order online at: **http://www.selfhealingmadeeasy.com** or complete & mail coupon.

## Please Print Clearly

Name _____

Address _____

City _____ State _____ Zip _____

Cell Phone _____ Home Phone _____

E-mail _____

*Please charge my*  ❏ Visa ❏ MC # _____

Exp. Date _____ $5.95 for Shipping & Handling

*Signature* _____

**Must have ALL the above info. No PO boxes please. No phone orders will be accepted.**

Mail this completed order form with check made out to:
**Angels to the Rescue, LLC, P.O. Box 2131, Bonita Springs, FL 34135**

Would you like to attend a ❏ Workshop or ❏ Private consultation by phone

Are you suffering for any particular condition? _____

What could you benefit from? _____